Cardiac Electrophysiology

A Visual Guide for Nurses, Techs, and Fellows

Second Edition

ONLINE ACCESS

The purchase of a new copy of this book entitles the first retail purchaser to free personal online access to a digital version of this edition.

Please send a copy of your purchase receipt to info@cardiotext.com with subject PURVES, 2ED EBOOK, and we will email you a redemption code along with instructions on how to access the digital file.

Cardiac Electrophysiology

A Visual Guide for Nurses, Techs, and Fellows

Second Edition

**Paul D. Purves, George J. Klein, Peter Leong-Sit,
Raymond Yee, Allan C. Skanes, Lorne J. Gula, Andrew D. Krahn**

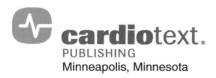

cardiotext.
PUBLISHING
Minneapolis, Minnesota

Second Edition

First Edition © 2012 Paul D. Purves
Second Edition © 2021 Paul D. Purves

Cardiotext Publishing, LLC
3405 W. 44th Street
Minneapolis, Minnesota 55410
USA
www.cardiotextpublishing.com

Any updates to this book may be found at:
www.cardiotextpublishing.com/electrophysiology-heart-rhythm-mgmt
/cardiac-electrophysiology-second-edition-purves

Comments, inquiries, and requests for bulk sales can be directed to the publisher
at: info@cardiotextpublishing.com.

Cover design by Paul D. Purves; interior design by Elizabeth Edwards

Library of Congress Control Number: 2020952895

ISBN: 978-1-942909-52-1
eISBN: 978-1-942909-53-8

Printed in Canada

1 2 3 4 5 6 7   25 24 23 22 21 21

Contents

continued

Contents *continued*

continued

Contents *continued*

About the Authors

Paul D. Purves, BSc, RCVT, CEPS

Senior Electrophysiology Technologist
Cardiac Investigation Unit
London Health Sciences Centre
London, Ontario, Canada

George J. Klein, MD, FRCP(C)

Professor of Medicine
Division of Cardiology
University of Western Ontario
London, Ontario, Canada

Peter Leong-Sit, MD, FRCP(C)

Assistant Professor of Medicine
Division of Cardiology
University of Western Ontario
London, Ontario, Canada

Raymond Yee, MD, FRCP(C)

Professor of Medicine
Director, Arrhythmia Service
Division of Cardiology
University of Western Ontario
London, Ontario, Canada

Allan C. Skanes, MD, FRCP(C)

Associate Professor of Medicine
Division of Cardiology
University of Western Ontario
London, Ontario, Canada

Lorne J. Gula, MD, FRCP(C)

Associate Professor of Medicine
Division of Cardiology
University of Western Ontario
London, Ontario, Canada

Andrew D. Krahn, MD, FRCP(C)

Professor of Medicine
Division of Cardiology
University of Western Ontario
London, Ontario, Canada

Foreword

The electrophysiology (EP) laboratory at the London Health Sciences Centre in London, Canada was established in 1980. Invasive EP was relatively new at that time and grew from groundbreaking innovations by key pioneers in several early centers of excellence. The ability to record electrograms from specific locations within the heart, including the His bundle, and to use programmed electrical stimulation of the heart to measure conduction parameters and induce arrhythmias was revolutionary. These advances amplified our ability to understand and treat cardiac rhythm disorders over and above what is possible with the electrocardiogram. The ensuing decades saw the introduction of more key innovations, including surgery for rhythm disorders, implantable devices, and most recently, catheter ablation.

Although the fundamental EP study is similar today to that performed in 1980, the broad range of enabling technologies available today has made it into a much more complex exercise requiring an equally broad range of skill sets and well-coordinated teamwork. "Teamwork" is not just a word when it comes to EP studies, where everyone's attention needs to be focused squarely on the job at hand. Because a single observation from any member of the team—nurse, technologist, physician assistant, or trainee—can make a critical difference in outcome, the entire team needs to be encouraged to stay involved and understand what is happening rather than just working in their little corner. No one should be afraid to present an observation to the team; in fact, we are all obligated to do so.

New trainees and personnel face a daunting challenge in acclimating to this setting! This may be especially true for technical and nursing staff who have little available to introduce them to the subject matter and the interpretation of the electrogram data in particular. Paul Purves is a unique EP technologist who has coupled his technical expertise and knowledge of EP with a passion for understanding the underpinnings of the study and teaches what he knows to other technologists, nurses, and indeed physicians. He is a gifted teacher who has coordinated and assembled the "collective wisdom" of our team into this reader-friendly and unique visual guide to performing and understanding the arrhythmia study. It surpasses the needs of a simple introduction and will be useful to all levels of trainee who want to understand what is really "going on" and move to the next level.

—*Dr. George J. Klein*

Preface

Cardiac Electrophysiology: A Visual Guide for Nurses, Techs, and Fellows is just that—a visual guide to electrophysiology. Written for allied health personnel, including nurses, technologists, industry personnel, and new EP fellows, this book presents the most important aspects of the EP study using pertinent images accompanied by detailed discussions of the principles involved. Topics covered include hardware connections ("connectology"), catheter placement, intracardiac signals, normal electrogram sequences associated with sinus rhythm, and—given an initial diagnosis of paroxysmal supraventricular tachycardia—the methodology we employ to uncover the mechanism of the tachycardia.

Because we have chosen to focus on the beginner, many complexities are either omitted or discussed in generalities only. The commentaries that follow most of the discussions throughout the book are intended to pique the reader's interest in advanced EP principles. Readers interested in gaining a more thorough understanding of these topics are referred to more comprehensive textbooks or to the current literature.

The computer/recording system used to generate the graphics in this guide may differ from the system with which you are familiar; however, the basic principles of signal processing (digitization, amplification, and filtering) remain the same. The channels displayed and their positions on the monitor are standard in our lab and may prove initially challenging if your lab organizes the display screen in a different manner. Regardless, try to focus on the information within these channels rather than on the cosmetics of how they are displayed. It is useful to interpret EP study findings no matter the format or from which center the recordings come, especially when preparing for EP certification examinations.

Teamwork in the EP lab is critical. In our lab, it is standard practice to encourage *everyone* to be involved and engaged in the diagnostic study and to be continually aware of any ECG changes, electrogram changes, or changes in catheter position. Checks and balances of this nature and a methodical, consistent approach are crucial components in the teamwork that enables any lab to run smoothly.

Acknowledgments

This textbook was initially inspired by my former cardiovascular technology student, Nicole Campbell—now my colleague—who correctly observed during her EP rotation that there was no textbook geared to her needs. It was also inspired by a constant stream of new cardiac arrhythmia fellows who similarly wanted a collection of tracings illustrating the basic concepts of electrophysiology. Thus was created a workbook and improved curriculum for my medical classroom. The workbook was expanded over the years and used more informally during the training of EP students across Canada. The physicians on our arrhythmia service and my coauthors are outstanding teachers and operate in an atmosphere of openness, mutual respect, and trust with their teammates. This collaborative environment allowed me to learn "on the job" as well as during invigorating arrhythmia rounds.

A special thanks to the great nurses and technologists with whom I have had the pleasure to work and who have had an unspoken impact on this effort:

Marilyn Braney, RN

Ellie Hogg, RCVT

Allena MacDonald, RN

Jane Schieman, RN

M.J. Vanstrien, RN

Thanks to my family—my wife Judy and daughters Mandy and Kelly—for their ongoing support and encouragement.

—*Paul D. Purves*

Video Descriptions

Abbreviations and Glossary

Accessory pathway

An additional electrical connection (other than the AV node) between the atria and ventricles

Accessory pathways may conduct:

- Antegrade only – generates a delta wave
- Retrograde only – no delta wave
- Bi-directional – generates a delta wave

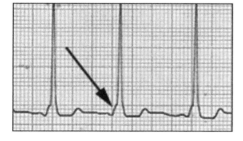

Action potential

The waveform generated by a cell's depolarization

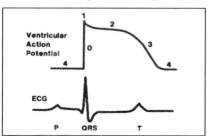

AEGM

Atrial electrogram

AF

Atrial fibrillation

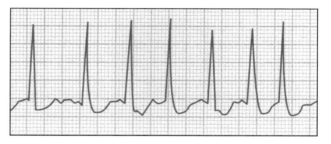

A-H interval

Transit time through the AV node

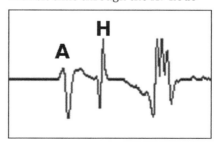

Anisotropy

The concept that conduction velocity is determined by the angle of initial depolarization

Antidromic

Denoting a wave of depolarization that is traveling retrogradely through the AV node. This term is usually used when describing the direction of the wavefront of an atrioventricular reentry circuit. In this scenario, the wave of depolarization travels down the accessory pathway and back up the AV node.

It can also denote a wave of depolarization that is traveling in the opposite direction to the predominate wave. For instance, a clockwise wave of depolarization introduced into a counterclockwise atrial flutter, therefore called an antidromic wavefront.

AP

Accessory pathway

Ashman's phenomenon

When a relatively long cycle (R-R) is followed by a relatively short R-R, the QRS associated with the short R-R often has right bundle branch block (RBBB) morphology. Often referred to a "long-shorting" the bundle branches. The right bundle branch has had insufficient time to adapt its ERP to a sudden change in heart rate. It therefore blocks.

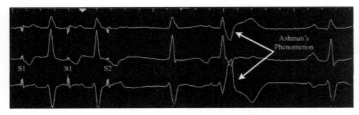

AT

Atrial tachycardia

Atrial fibrillation

A disorganized atrial rhythmrhythm (see AF above)

Atropine

A parasympatholytic used to increase heart rate

AV

Referring to the atrioventricular node or atrioventricular conduction

AVCS

AV conduction system

AVNRT

AV nodal reentrant tachycardia

AVRT

Atrioventricular reentrant tachycardia

Bipolar

Refers to the use of two poles (a positive and a negative electrode), usually in close proximity to one another. However, a unipolar lead is just a widely spaced bipole.

Bundle of His

Anatomic structure connecting the AV node to the bundle branches

Carto

A 3D mapping system from Biosense Webster

CFEs

Complex fractionated electrograms, usually associated with the left atrium during AF

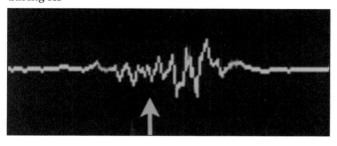

Chevron

CS 1-2 activation occurs as early as CS 9-10 activation

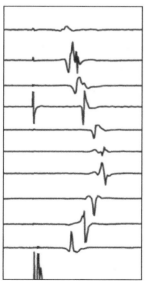

Concealed

An unseen penetration of a wave of depolarization into a structure that subsequently affects the conduction properties of that structure

Contralateral

On the other side – it often is used as "contralateral bundle branch block"

It refers to:

- a LBBB pattern during a right-sided tachycardia
- a RBBB during a left-sided tachycardia
- the effect of that bundle branch block on the tachycardia

CS

Coronary sinus

CTI

Cavo-tricuspid isthmus

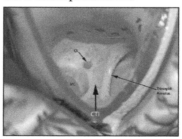

Decapolar

A 10-pole catheter, often the CS catheter

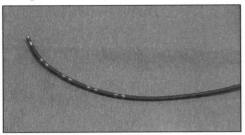

Decrement

The ability of the AV node to slow conduction

Delta wave

The initial part of this widened QRS that represents conduction directly into the ventricle

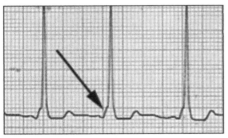

Depolarization

The process by which a cell changes on the inside from electrically negative to electrically positive

Digitization

The conversion of an analog signal to a digital signal

Duo-deca

A 20-pole catheter

ECG

Electrocardiogram

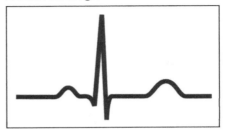

Echo

An unexpected return of a wave of depolarization to the chamber where the wave originated

EGM

Electrogram

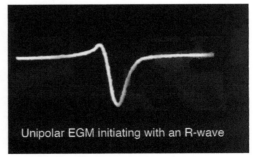

Unipolar EGM initiating with an R-wave

Entrainment

A pacing maneuver where we pace slightly faster than the tachycardia cycle length, temporarily speed up the tachycardia circuit, then stop pacing to allow the circuit to return to its initial cycle length. The main purpose to determine how close to the tachycardia circuit the pacing catheter is.

EP

Electrophysiology

ERP

Effective refractory period – the longest S1S2 that fails to conduct. Most of the time we are looking for the ERP of the AV node or an accessory pathway. With a very tight S1S2 (600, 200), you may reach the ERP of the myocardium itself (seen as no capture of the S2).

FP

AV nodal fast pathway

FRP

Functional refractory period

Examples:

- Referring to the AV node, it is the shortest output (H1-H2) achievable in response to any S1S2 input, which means that no decrement has occurred yet
- Referring to the ventricle, it is the shortest V1-V2 achievable from any S1S2 input, which means no latency has occurred yet

Gap

An unexpected resumption of conduction after block has occurred

HIS

The connecting cable between AV node and bundle branches

His-Purkinje system

The specialized conduction system within the ventricles

HRA

High right atrium/high right atrial

H-V interval

Transit time from the His bundle to the ventricle

Ipsilateral

On the same side – it often is used as "ipsilateral bundle branch block." It refers to a RBBB pattern during a right-sided tachycardia or a LBBB during a left-sided tachycardia and the effect of that bundle branch block on the tachycardia.

Isoproterenol

Isuprel – a sympathomimetic. Used to increase heart rate and used in the EP lab to alter autonomic tone in the AV node.

Jump

A sudden lengthening of the V-A time or A-V time of 50 msec or more with a tightening of the S2 coupling interval of 10 msec. A sudden, abrupt prolongation of the A-H interval.

Junctional

Beats that originate from the junctional region below the AV node

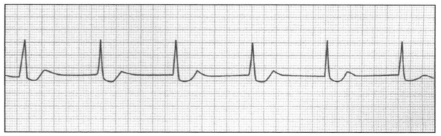

LAH

Left anterior hemiblock. Lead 1 is positive. Lead 2 is negative.

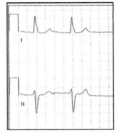

LAO

Left anterior oblique

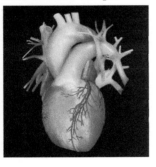

Lasso

A duo-decapolar catheter and the trademark name for a circular mapping catheter (Biosense Webster)

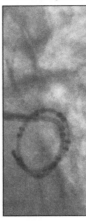

Latency

The time period between delivery of the pacing stimulus and the local depolarization of the myocardium

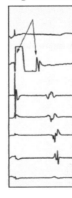

LBBB
Left bundle branch block

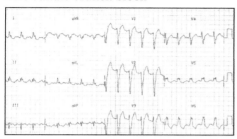

LCP
Lower common pathway

LPH
Left posterior hemiblock. Lead 1 is negative. Lead 2 is positive.

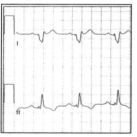

LRA
Low right atrium/low right atrial

MRA
Mid right atrium/mid right atrial

NC
No capture

Orthodromic
Denoting a wave of depolarization that is traveling antegradely through the AV node. Also a wave of depolarization traveling in the same direction as the predominant wavefront.

Overdrive suppression
When another focus within the heart spontaneously depolarizes faster than the SA node, the SA node is effectively put to sleep. Since the SA node drives a heart rate of 70 beats per minute and the junction drives the heart rate at 40 beats per minute, the SA node "overdrive suppresses" the junction. Similarly, a junctional escape rhythm of 40 beats per minute will overdrive suppress a ventricular escape rhythm of 20 beats per minute.

PAC
Premature atrial contraction

P-A interval
Transatrial conduction time

Para-Hisian pacing
Refers to pacing beside or close to the bundle of His (para = beside or next to). A pacing maneuver used to determine the presence or absence of an antero-septal accessory pathway.

Paroxysmal
Usually used as a descriptor of atrial fibrillation that lasts only a few hours and may be used with any tachycardia lasting only a few hours

Persistent
Atrial fibrillation lasting days or longer

PPI
Post-pacing interval

Pre-excitation
Ventricular activation via an accessory pathway

PR interval
The timing between the onset of the P-wave and the onset of the QRS

PV
Pulmonary vein

PVC
Premature ventricular contraction

P wave
Atrial depolarization on the ECG

QRS
Ventricular depolarization on the ECG

Radiofrequency
The type of energy delivered to ablate cardiac tissue (the frequency is 350–500 kHz)

RAO
Right anterior oblique

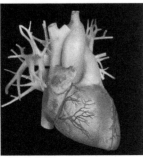

RBBB
Right bundle branch block

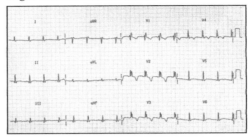

Refractory
Denoting a time when the tissue is unresponsive to electrical stimulation

RVA
Right ventricular apex

S1
Stimulus 1; the drive train of 8 beats

S2
Stimulus 2; the first extra-stimulus after the drive train

S3
Stimulus 3; the second extra-stimulus after the drive train

SA
Sino-atrial

SP
AV nodal slow pathway

Spontaneous normalization

The ability of either bundle branch to adapt its conduction properties and thus transition from a LBBB or RBBB pattern to a normal QRS morphology

SVT

Supraventricular tachycardia

Tachycardia

Rapid heart rate, usually more than 100 beats per minute

TCL

Tachycardia cycle length

Transseptal conduction

Refers to a wave of depolarization conducting across the interventricular septum. It can be from RV to LV or LV to RV. Such myocardial conduction is much slower than conduction through the specialized bundle branch system.

T wave

Ventricular repolarization on the ECG

Unipolar

Refers to the use of a single pole (by convention, the positive electrode) in contact with the area of interest and a distant second electrode (by convention, the negative electrode). In essence, it is a VERY widely spaced bipole.

V-A

Ventriculo-atrial

V-A interval

Conduction time from ventricle to atrium

VEGM

Ventricular electrogram

VERP

Ventricular effective refractory period

VF

Ventricular fibrillation

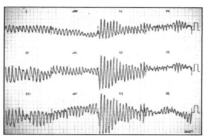

VT

Ventricular tachycardia

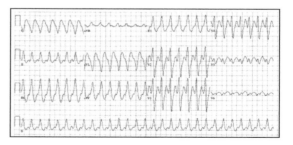

Wenckebach

The pacing interval at which a loss of 1:1 conduction between the atria and the ventricles occurs

WPW
Wolff-Parkinson-White (syndrome)

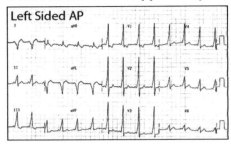

Before We Begin an SVT Study

There are many reasons for patients to undergo an electrophysiology (EP) procedure. However, not every patient needs a full diagnostic study for supraventricular tachycardia (SVT), which involves incremental ventricular pacing followed by ventricular extra-stimulus pacing, atrial extra-stimulus pacing, and finally, atrial incremental pacing. Rather, the choice of catheters and equipment will change depending on the intent of the procedure. When the diagnosis has been clearly established, a more focused approach is employed. For example, if typical atrial flutter is the working diagnosis, our study will be abbreviated and focused as follows:

1. Confirm, using entrainment, that it is indeed a typical, cavo-tricuspid isthmus (CTI)–dependent flutter.

2. Proceed with a CTI ablation.

By contrast, if atrial fibrillation (AF) is the confirmed diagnosis, the diagnostic portion of the study will be very minimal to absent, and the ablation will be started after the appropriate setup.

The catheter setup and diagnostic techniques employed are unique and specific to the situation, but the SVT study forms the model for all studies and will be presented in more detail as such in the text to follow.

Before We Begin an SVT Study *continued*

In this example, the clinical diagnosis was unclear so a full diagnostic study was performed. AV nodal reentrant tachycardia (AVNRT) was the final diagnosis. Remember, just because the patient demonstrates AVNRT does not eliminate the possibility that a substrate for a different tachycardia (eg, accessory pathway [AP]) exists. Our full diagnostic study ruled this out.

Commentary: Entrainment (mentioned on page 1) is covered later in this guide.

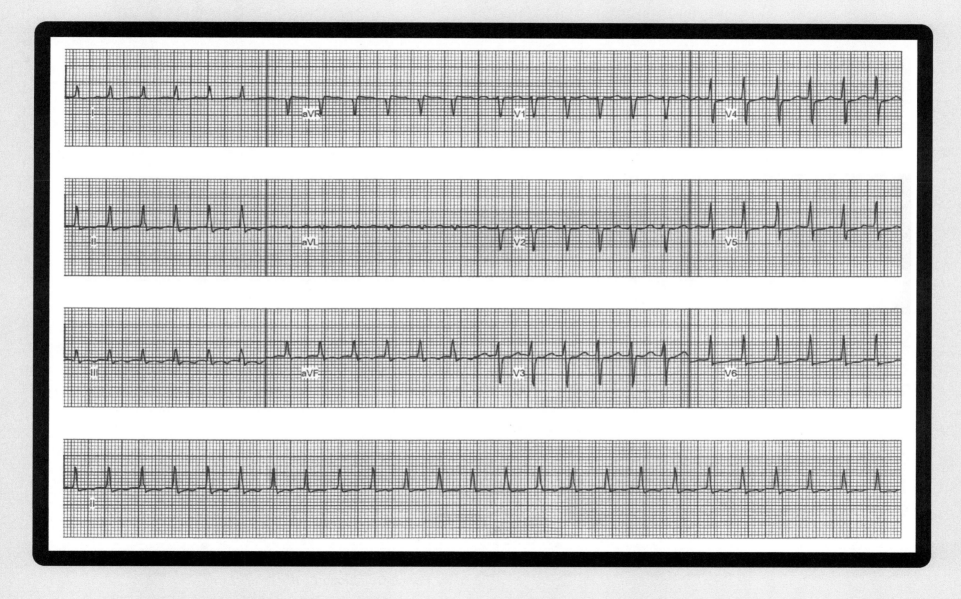

Unit 1:
The Basics

In this unit we look at catheter placement, the computer system, signal processing, signal sequence in sinus rhythm, basic conduction intervals, and two basic but critical tissue characteristics:

- Conduction velocity
- Refractoriness

Understanding these concepts is critical to understanding the mechanisms of most tachycardias.

Starting on page 18, you will find our methodology and the sequence of cardiac stimulation we use in a routine diagnostic study for SVT. Examining the normal sequence of signal conduction and measuring various basic intervals establishes a baseline for the patient. These measurements will vary depending on the clinical problem.

UNIT 1 OUTLINE

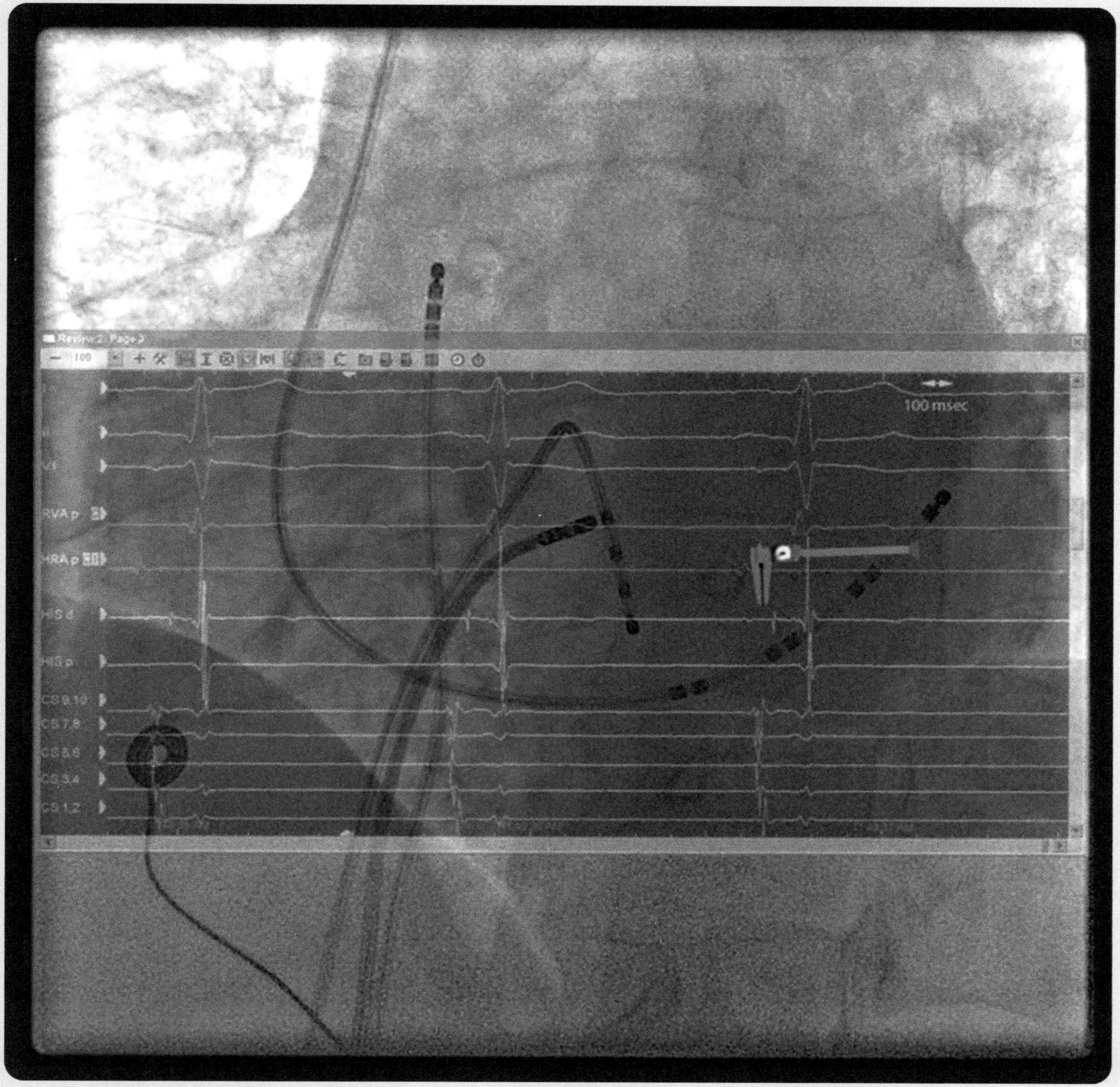
100 msec
V1
RVA p
HRA p
HIS d
HIS p
CS 9,10
CS 7,8
CS 5,6
CS 3,4
CS 1,2

1. Catheter Placement

Multi-electrode catheters are exclusively used in clinical EP. Electrical signals are detected and recorded from the individual electrodes and from adjacent electrodes (bipole). By convention, the most distal electrode (at the tip of the catheter) is numbered 1. Subsequent electrodes are numbered in a sequential fashion, as shown in the coronary sinus (CS) decapolar catheter here (labeled in green).

The high right atrial (HRA) catheter is labeled in red. It will record an atrial (A) signal on the red HRA channel on our tracings throughout this book. The HIS catheter is labeled in yellow. It is positioned in the region of the atrioventricular (AV) node guided by both the signals and fluoroscopic images. Since the AV node is in close proximity to both the atria and the ventricles, it will have both an A signal as well as a ventricular (V) signal. In addition, the HIS catheter will have a third electrogram (EGM) representing the bundle of His, which is the electrical conduit from the AV node to the specialized conduction system within the ventricles. This EGM is often referred to simply as an "H." So the properly positioned HIS catheter will display three EGMs—atrial (A), HIS (H), and ventricular (V)—on our yellow HIS channel. The right ventricular apex (RVA) catheter is labeled in magenta. It will display a V signal on our magenta RVA channel.

The CS catheter is labeled in green. The CS is the vein situated between the left atrium and the left ventricle. Therefore, this catheter, for the most part, identifies signals from the left atrium and left ventricle when properly positioned within the CS. It is our custom that CS 9-10 should be positioned at the left edge of the spine in the left anterior oblique (LAO) projection. This "neutral" position places these poles at the junction of the right atrium and the CS opening. CS 1-2 will display signals from the lateral aspect of the left atrium. Most CS signals will have two components, A and V, on our green CS channel. Currently, we use a 10-pole (decapolar) CS catheter.

Commentary: Atrial activation sequence proceeds from proximal to distal in the normal heart assuming a normally positioned (neutral or central) CS catheter. If the CS catheter is not in the neutral position, atrial activation during ventricular pacing may appear eccentric and thus be very misleading (ie, mimicking APs). If the CS catheter is advanced too far into the CS, the signals may appear as a chevron (ie, CS 1-2 activation is as early as CS 9-10 activation). This early activation is due to detection of Bachmann's bundle.

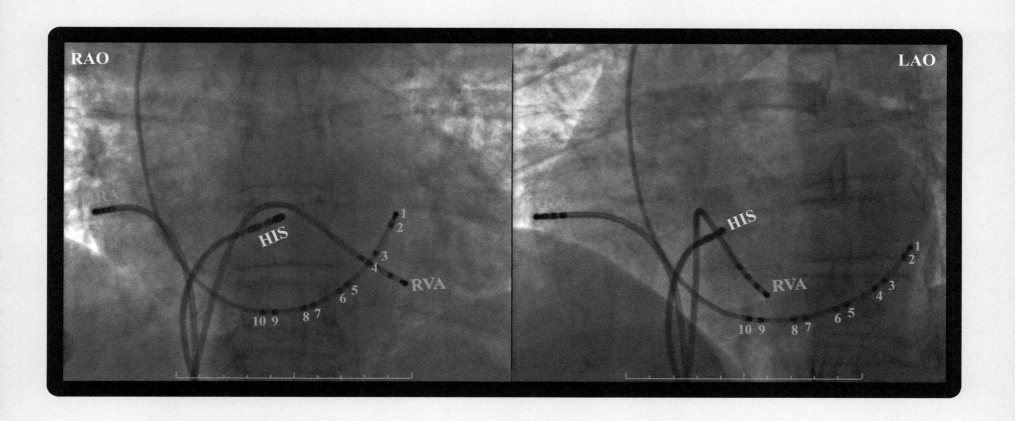

2. The Computer System

All intracardiac catheters are plugged into patient interface blocks via connecting cables. The electrical signals detected from the catheters are sent to these blocks. From here, the signals are sent to the amplifier and then on to the recording system and monitors.

How your computer/recording system displays these signals is quite customizable. The colors of individual EGMs, signal location on the screen, order of the catheters displayed on the screen, gains, and filters are entirely modifiable.

In this image, we have our CS catheter plugged into the interface block on the far right. To see these signals, we instruct the computer to display Block A >> pins 1 to 10 >> and color them green. We then position these bipole signals (CS 1-2, CS 3-4, CS 5-6, CS 7-8, CS 9-10) at the bottom of our screen.

When troubleshooting, keep in mind that problems often stem from a "connectology" issue. Be sure catheters are connected securely to the connection cables, cables to the interface boxes, and boxes to the amplifier. Also check that channel gains are appropriate, filters have not been changed, and someone didn't turn off the signal display. It is not uncommon to accidentally plug the catheters into the wrong pins on these blue interface boxes and thus display no signals at all.

Commentary: Filtering of signals is explained in greater detail on page 10.

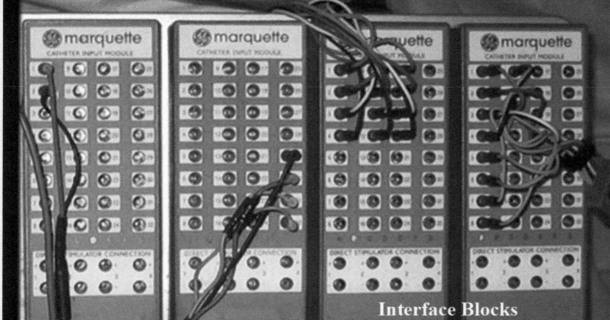

Connecting Cables

Interface Blocks

Connections to Amp, Recording system and Monitors

3. Signal Processing

How we see the signals on the monitor is a result of various processing procedures. You need to understand the concepts of gain, clipping, high-pass filters, and low-pass filters. This image shows the settings for electrocardiogram (ECG) filtering (channels 1–12) and three intracardiac channel settings (channels 33–48).

Gain simply increases the amplitude, or size, of the signal. It only amplifies whatever is on that channel, including (unfortunately) noise. Clipping is simply constraining the size of a signal to a geographic location on the monitor such that two adjacent signals don't overlap each other.

High-pass and low-pass filters are often confused. The high-pass filter allows any signals higher than the preset frequency (Hz) to be passed through to the monitor. Therefore, it filters out low-frequency signals, such as a wandering baseline. In this example, any intracardiac signal with a frequency higher than 30 Hz will be allowed to pass through to the monitor and any signal lower than 30 Hz will be blocked. The low-pass filter allows any signals less than the preset frequency to be passed through to the monitor. It, therefore, filters out high-frequency signals. In this example, any intracardiac signal with a frequency lower than 500 Hz will be allowed to pass through to the monitor and any signal higher than 500 Hz will be blocked.

The total effect is to allow signals between 30 and 500 Hz to be displayed. Signals outside this range are blocked from view.

The notch pass is a special and a relatively specific 60-Hz noise filter.

Commentary: Changing the high-pass filter on the ECG can markedly change its morphology. Try it and see the result. Highly filtered signals look "cleaner" but remove information, possibly important information. There is always a compromise between obtaining a clean signal and maintaining the information required. The filter settings displayed here are nominal and consistent across most recording systems.

Channel	Label	Gain	Filter Settings		Notch Pass	Active
			High Pass	Low Pass		
1	I	10000	0.50 Hz	100 Hz	On	On
2	II	2500	0.50 Hz	100 Hz	On	On
3	III	2500	0.50 Hz	100 Hz	On	On
4	aVR	2500	0.50 Hz	100 Hz	On	On
5	aVL	2500	0.50 Hz	100 Hz	On	On
6	aVF	2500	0.50 Hz	100 Hz	On	On
7	V1	5000	0.50 Hz	100 Hz	On	On
8	V2	2500	0.50 Hz	100 Hz	On	On
9	V3	2500	0.50 Hz	100 Hz	On	On
10	V4	2500	0.50 Hz	100 Hz	On	On
11	V5	2500	0.50 Hz	100 Hz	On	On
12	V6	2500	0.50 Hz	100 Hz	On	On

Channel	Label	Type	Inputs		Gain	Filter Settings		Notch Pass
			+	-		High Pass	Low Pass	
33	RVa d	Bipolar	2	1	2500	30.00 Hz	500 Hz	
34	RVa p	Bipolar	4	3	2500	30.00 Hz	500 Hz	
35	HIS d	Bipolar	10	9	10000	30.00 Hz	500 Hz	
36	HIS p	Bipolar	12	11	5000	30.00 Hz	500 Hz	
37	HRA d	Bipolar	18	17	5000	30.00 Hz	500 Hz	
38	HRA p	Bipolar	20	19	5000	30.00 Hz	500 Hz	
39		Not Used						
40		Not Used						
41		Not Used						
42		Not Used						
43		Not Used						
44		Not Used						
45		Not Used						
46		Not Used						
47	Stim 3	Stim 3			250	30.00 Hz	500 Hz	On
48	Stim 4	Stim 4			250	30.00 Hz	500 Hz	On

4. Signal Sequence in Sinus Rhythm

1st: The HRA A electrogram (AEGM) is the earliest since this catheter is closest to the sino-atrial (SA) node. Note that it corresponds to the onset of the surface P-wave.

2nd: HIS A is the next AEGM to appear in sequence. The wave of atrial depolarization has successfully arrived at the AV node.

3rd: CS A signals appear next as the wave spreads from the proximal CS distally into the left atrium.

4th: The H deflection on the HIS catheter is next. This indicates that the wave has propagated over the atrioventricular (AV) node and arrived at the bundle of His.

5th: The RVA V electrogram (VEGM) is generally next as it is near to the right bundle branch exit, which is usually the first part of the ventricles to be activated. Note that it is before the HIS V or CS V signals since the wave of depolarization travels down the bundle branches, past the apex, and arrives at the base of the ventricles last.

6th: The HIS channel V and the CS V's are the last signals to occur. Remember that the HIS and CS catheters are positioned at the base of the ventricles.

Commentary: Take careful note that the RVA V signal is ahead of the HIS V and CS V signals in sinus rhythm since the right ventricle is activated early in normal depolarization without bundle branch block. On the other hand, the HIS or CS V signal may precede the right ventricle with right bundle branch block (RBBB), where the left ventricle will be activated before the right. This relationship could change if an AP is present and may give a clue as to the insertion site of the AP into the ventricles.

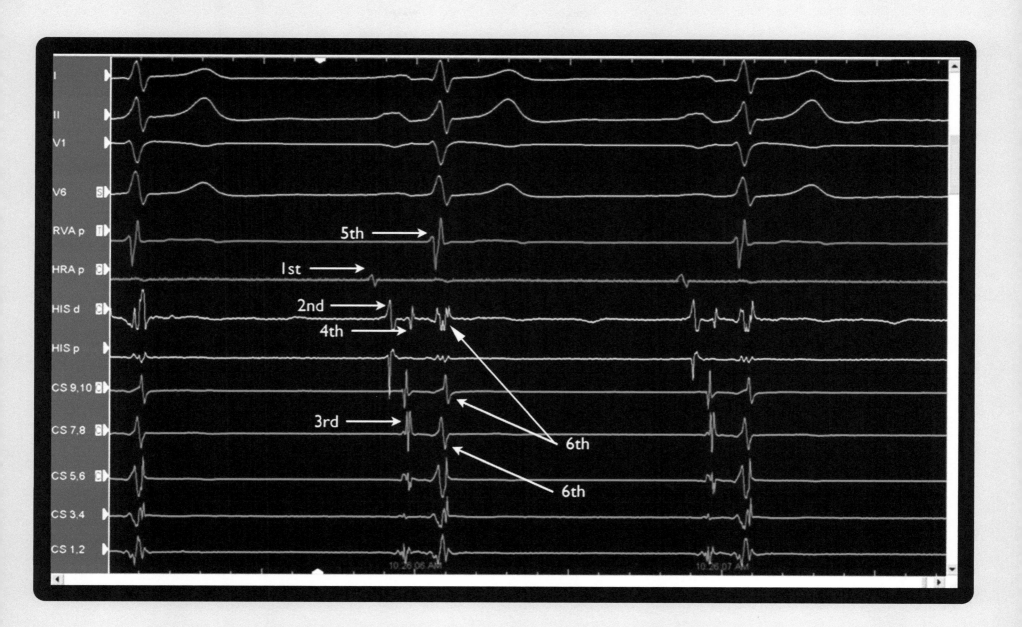

5. Basic Conduction Intervals

Routine baseline measurements should be made and recorded for every patient undergoing an EP study. The names and normal ranges are as follows:

- **P-A interval**: Measure from the onset of the P-wave on the surface ECG to the rapid deflection of the A-wave on the HIS channel. (See the red calipers.) The P-A interval is usually about 35 to 45 msec. This is the transright atrial conduction time, that is, the approximate time it takes for the electrical signal to travel from the SA node to the AV node.

- **A-H interval**: Measure on the HIS channel as the A signal to the onset of the H deflection. (See the white calipers.) The A-H interval is usually about 70 to 80 msec. This is the transnodal conduction time, or the time it takes for the electrical signal to travel through the AV node.

- **H-V interval**: Measure from the onset of the HIS deflection to the earliest onset of ventricular activation on any channel available, either intracardiac or ECG. (See the green calipers.) It is usually the onset of the QRS complex. The H-V interval is about 35 to 45 msec. This is the His to ventricular activation time, that is, the time it takes for the electrical signal to travel from the His bundle to the ventricles.

Therefore, on a surface ECG, these three measurements make up the PR interval:

$$\textbf{PR interval} = \text{P-A} + \text{A-H} + \text{H-V}$$
$$= 40 + 80 + 40$$
$$= 160 \text{ msec}$$

Commentary: Careful measurement of these basic intervals is critical. You must know the baseline A-H in order to recognize subsequent AV nodal decrement and potential "jumps." Additionally, a long H-V interval indicates distal His-Purkinje disease.

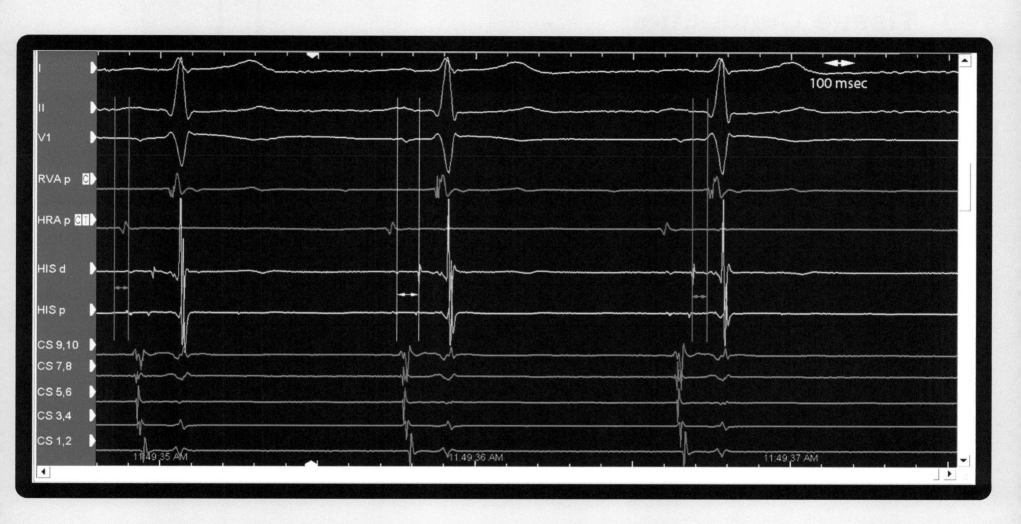

6. Tissue Conduction

The key concepts to understand about tissue conduction are:

- Tissue conduction velocity
- Refractoriness

Tissue conduction velocity refers to the speed at which the electrical signals travel between cells in a specific part of the heart. In contrast, the refractory period measures recovery time of the tissue before it can conduct electrical signals again.

Tissues with rapid conduction time may or may not have short refractory periods and vice versa. The usual measurement we cite is the effective refractory period (ERP). For example, the ERP of the AV node is the longest atrial extra-stimulus (or A1-A2) that *fails* to conduct to the His bundle as the extra-stimuli are gradually decremented, that is, brought progressively closer to the last paced beat (last A signal of the eight-beat drive cycle). Another common measure that also essentially gauges refractoriness is the block cycle length. The block cycle length is determined via incremental pacing (pacing progressively faster in small increments) and is the longest cycle that blocks. This is usually referred to as the Wenckebach cycle length. A short block cycle length indicates tissue capable of sustaining rapid rates during a tachycardia.

Commentary: This image is a schematic illustration of the extra-stimulus technique using the example of an atrial stimulation site. Time is represented horizontally, and the passage of the impulse through the heart is represented vertically. The heart is paced at a defined rate (generally eight beats), designated S1. In successive runs, an extra-stimulus (S2) is made progressively more premature to the last S1 and thus "scans" the cardiac cycle. S2 is progressively decreased until it fails to capture the atrium.

The top row shows a drive with conduction occurring over a "fast" AV nodal pathway. The second row shows block of the impulse at the fast pathway with conduction over the "slow" AV nodal pathway. In the third row, the S2 is sufficiently premature to block to the slow pathway. The fourth row shows an S2 that is sufficiently premature to prevent atrial capture. In this way, the ERPs of the various structures can be determined (ie, the longest coupling interval that doesn't make it to the next level).

A = conduction through the atrium, AVCS = AV conduction system,
V = conduction in the ventricle, FP = fast pathway, SP = slow pathway,
NC = no capture (the atrial ERP)

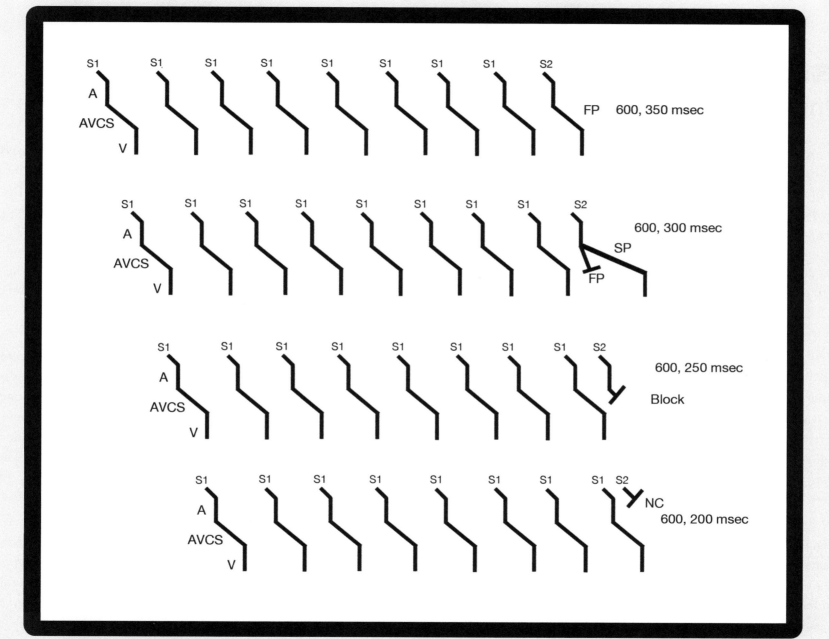

7. Supraventricular Tachycardia Diagnostic Study
Incremental Ventricular Pacing

Our diagnostic study begins with incremental ventricular pacing to establish the retrograde block cycle length (Wenckebach cycle length) of the A-V conduction system. Pacing begins 100 msec faster than the patient's intrinsic rate and decreases by 10 to 20 msec every eight beats until 1:1 ventriculo-atrial (V-A) conduction is no longer maintained. We do not pace faster than 250 msec because ventricular tachycardia (VT) or ventricular fibrillation (VF) may be induced at higher rates. There are four basic questions to consider:

1. **Did the pacing capture the ventricle?** Inspect the ECG and EGMs to confirm that the pacing stimulus did indeed capture the ventricle.

2. **Is there V-A conduction?** Look at the RVA channel (magenta) and the HRA channel (red) and establish the relationship between ventricular activation and atrial activation. This example shows each VEGM followed by an AEGM, or 1:1 conduction (*arrows*). At any given pacing rate, there may be no V-A conduction at all (the A signals will have no relationship to the V signals) or there may be V-A conduction that is 2:1 or some other ratio.

3. **What is the pattern of retrograde atrial activation?** In the normal heart, retrograde conduction to the atrium occurs via the AV node so that atrial activation will occur here first. This is referred to as "central" or "concentric" atrial activation and is seen as the yellow HIS A being the first A seen following the large V. It is generally slightly ahead of any CS A. The proximal CS is close to the AV node and is thus activated next. That is, the CS AEGMs activate at CS 7-8 first, followed by CS 5-6, CS 3-4, and finally CS 1-2. This central pattern is the expected pattern when retrograde conduction is through the AV node. When the earliest A signal is not at the HIS A, the pattern is referred to as "eccentric" atrial activation, which suggests that there may be another connection between the ventricles and the atrium other than the AV node (ie, an AP).

4. **Does the V-A time stay constant or become prolonged (decrements) as we increase the pacing rate?** The expected behavior of the AV node is that conduction slows at higher pacing rates. Therefore, at higher rates, the V-A time should be longer if conduction is going through the AV node (due to its decremental properties). This is readily obvious on the CS channels. Most APs do not decrement. Therefore, the absence of V-A time prolongation at higher pacing rates suggests conduction using an AP.

Commentary: The fifth question is "What is the V-A time?" A long V-A time could indicate a retrograde slow pathway or a decremental AP. Since both demonstrate a long V-A time, making an accurate diagnosis of the tachycardia circuit may be quite challenging! More pacing maneuvers are required.

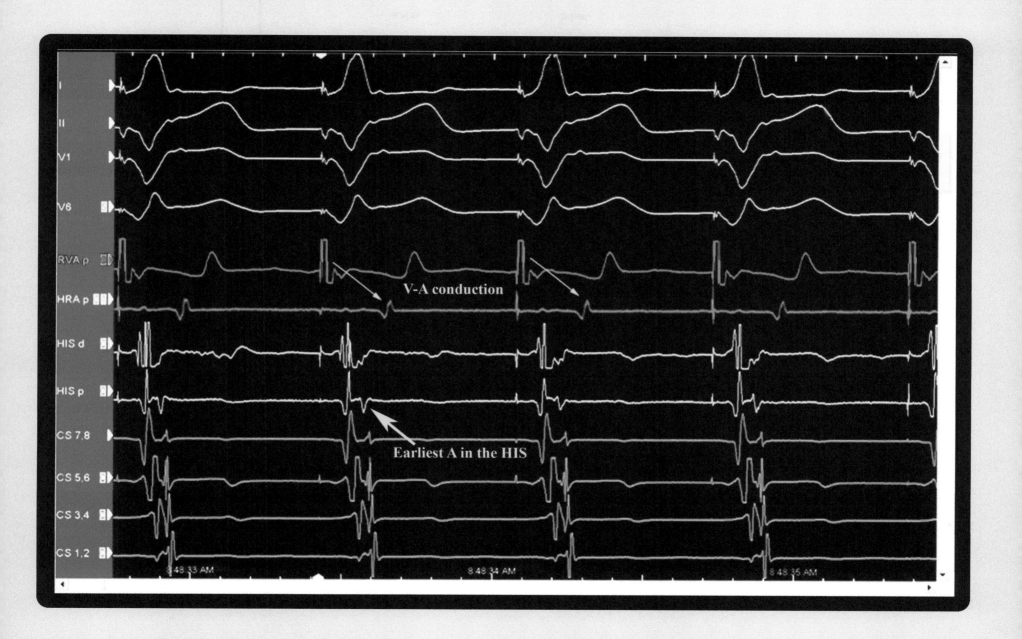

7. Supraventricular Tachycardia Diagnostic Study *continued*
Retrograde Wenckebach

This tracing illustrates the loss of 1:1 V-A conduction. The pacing interval at which this occurs is referred to as the retrograde block cycle length or the retrograde Wenckebach point.

Notice that the V capture in the magenta RVA channel is followed by a red A in the HRA channel for the first three paced beats. The fourth paced beat (*third arrow*) shows a magenta V but no associated red A. This loss of an HRA A signal confirms that we have reached the Wenckebach point of the retrograde A-V conduction system.

Also notice in the yellow HIS and green CS channels that the time from the V signal to the A signal has lengthened compared with the tracing on the previous page, implying decrement in the AV node as we increase our pacing rate. The level of block with incremental pacing is generally at the AV node.

This is normal AV nodal physiology.

Commentary: A common mistake is not appreciating minimal decrement. You must measure the V-A time at the beginning of this pacing maneuver and monitor throughout the run as well as at the end. You measure a V-A time from the onset of ventricular activation to the earliest A signal on any channel. Absence of decrement may be seen with the normal V-A conduction system but should raise the suspicion of an AP (Wolff-Parkinson-White [WPW] syndrome).

▶ Video 1.1: **Incremental V Pacing**

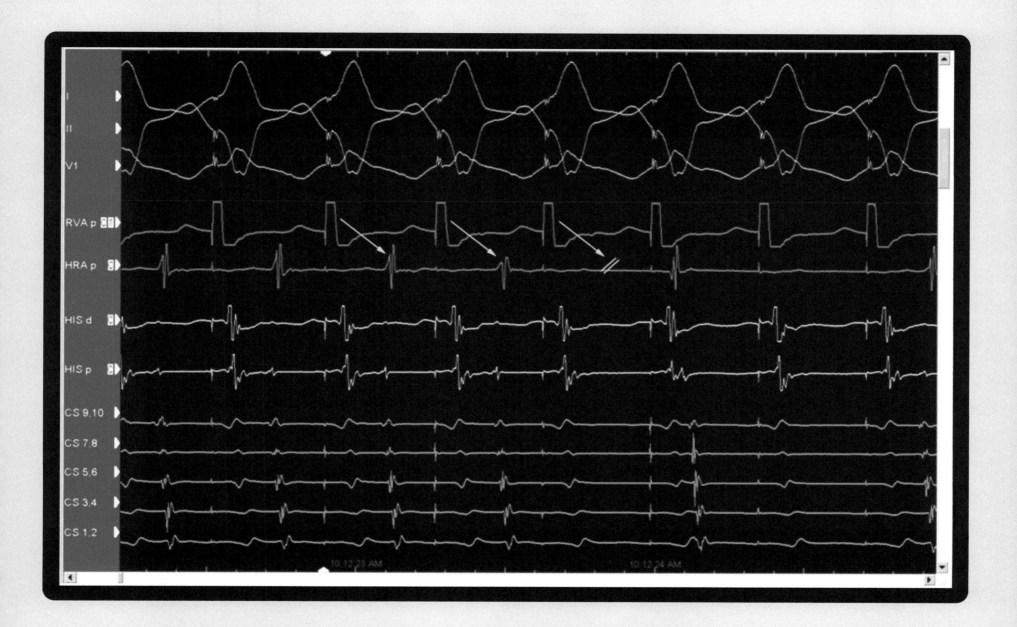

7. Supraventricular Tachycardia Diagnostic Study *continued*
Ventricular Extra-stimulus Pacing

This pacing sequence frequently induces the culprit clinical tachycardia in addition to establishing the conduction properties of the retrograde conduction system. An extra-systole (S2) is introduced after a drive train of eight S1s. The timing between the last S1 and the S2 is known as the S1-S2 coupling interval, and this is progressively decreased with each pacing sequence.

We generally do two runs at different drive cycle lengths, usually 600 and 400 msec. For example, at a drive train of 600, the coupling intervals are 600-580, 600-560...600-200 msec.

We do a second drive train with coupling intervals of 400-380, 400-360...400-200 msec. Be aware that there is no consistent relationship between antegrade and retrograde conduction over the A-V conduction system or indeed any other cardiac tissue.

As one shortens the S1-S2 coupling interval, the V-A conduction time following the S2 will lengthen, usually due to decrement in the AV node. This can be clearly seen on the CS channels following the S2 in this example.

Commentary: You may note a sudden lengthening of the V-A interval during this procedure (>50 msec). This sudden lengthening of the V-A time is frequently referred to as a "jump" and suggests a change in the retrograde conduction pathway. This may be due to:

- Conduction block in the retrograde fast AV nodal pathway switching to a retrograde slow pathway in the AV node
- Conduction block in an AP switching to conduction over the AV node or vice versa
- Retrograde block in the right bundle branch, followed by transseptal conduction and conduction up the left bundle. This will delay retrograde His bundle activation as well give us a retrograde HIS deflection. See page 136.

▶ Video 1.2: **V Extra-stimulus Pacing**

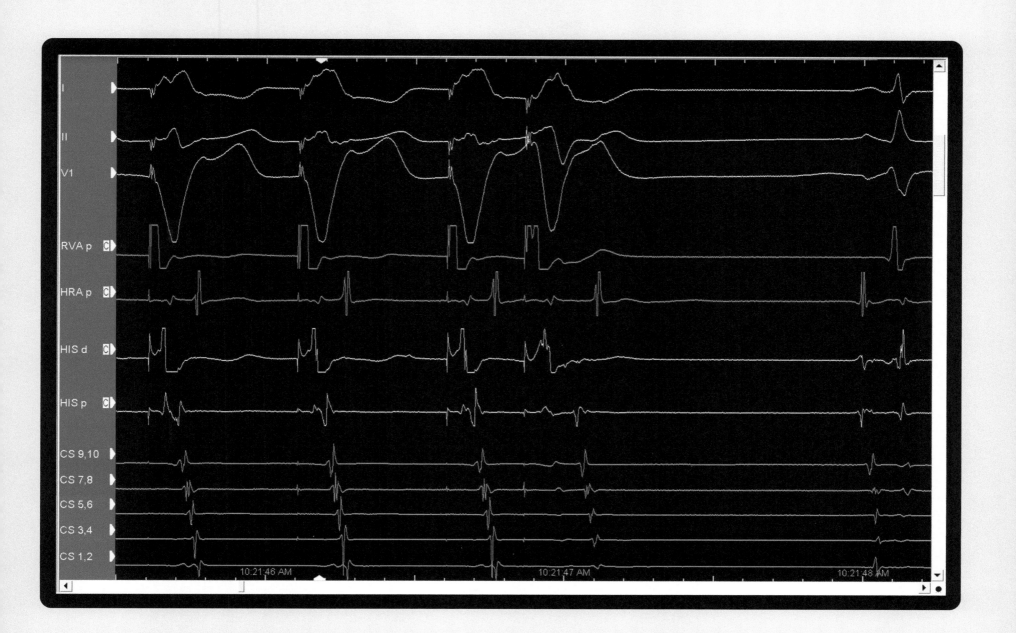

7. Supraventricular Tachycardia Diagnostic Study *continued*
Retrograde V-A block

As we continue to shorten the S1-S2 coupling interval, we reach the point at which V-A conduction fails to conduct to the atrium since it has not had sufficient time to recover after conducting the last S1. We have thus reached the retrograde ERP of the V-A conduction system (usually due to block in the AV node).

In this tracing, note that the magenta S2 is *not* followed by a red A on the HRA channel (*third arrow*). We document this as V-A conduction block. This is also apparent from a lack of A signals on the other channels.

V-A conduction is quite variable from individual to individual. It may be completely absent or the retrograde ERP may be very short.

As mentioned earlier, some individuals have two retrograde pathways over the AV node, one with fast conduction and one with slow conduction. We may see the V-A time suddenly "jump" from a short V-A time to a much longer V-A time, possibly reflecting the switch from the fast to the slow pathway. This jump should be noted and may suggest the substrate for a reentrant circuit.

Commentary: Once we have reached the ERP of the V-A conducting system, we continue to shorten the S1-S2 coupling interval until the stimulus fails to capture the ventricle. Paradoxically, nodal conduction may resume at a shorter coupling interval. This is known as "gap phenomenon" and is described on page 104.

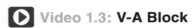 Video 1.3: **V-A Block**

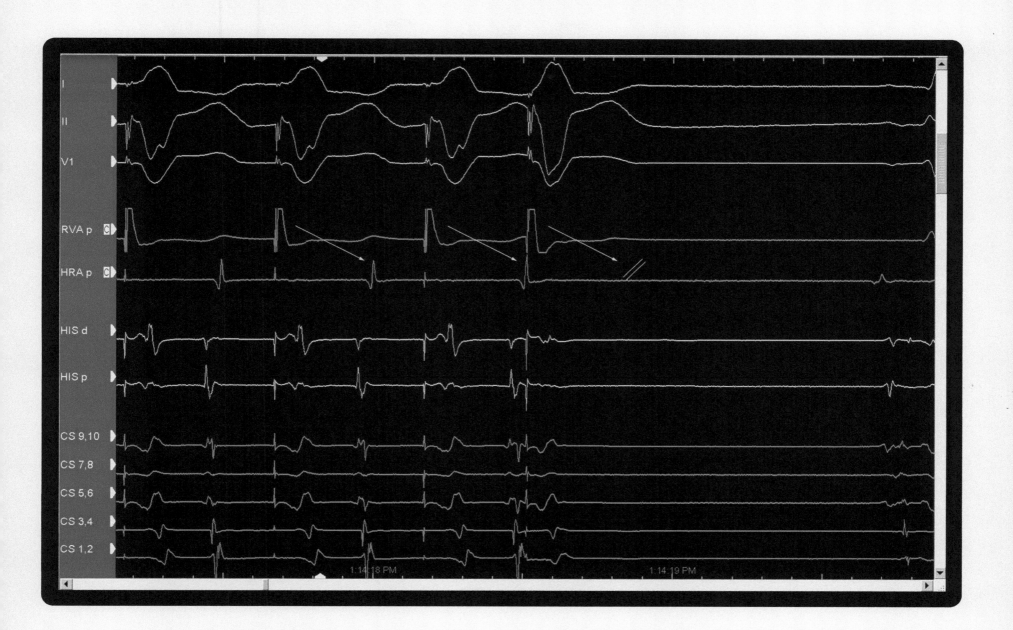

7. Supraventricular Tachycardia Diagnostic Study *continued*
Ventricular Effective Refractory Period

As we shorten the S1-S2 coupling interval, we reach the point at which the myocardium itself can no longer respond to the S2 since it is still refractory from the previous S1. We have now reached the ERP of the ventricular myocardium.

We document this as "no capture" (NC) or ventricular effective refractory period (VERP). Note that the S2 pacing artifact or "spike" (as seen on the surface ECG or the magenta RVA channel) does not generate a QRS on the surface ECG. Be sure that this is truly NC, as this loss of capture may also be caused by catheter movement inside the heart with failure to make contact with the myocardium. If you are unsure, repeat the drive and coupling interval to confirm that the NC is reproducible.

NC typically occurs with the S2 coupling interval in range of 250 to 200 msec.

Commentary: NC can also occur due to an insufficient pacing current. Before the study begins, you must establish the pacing threshold for the atria and the ventricles. The study is generally conducted while pacing at two or three times this threshold. Typically, if the catheters are positioned securely, both atria and ventricles will capture at 2 mA and a pulse width of 2 msec. The CS catheter, being along the A-V ring, may capture either the atrium (usually more proximally) or the ventricle (more distally in CS). The CS catheter typically needs more current to capture either the atrium or the ventricle due to poorer tissue contact.

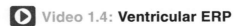 Video 1.4: **Ventricular ERP**

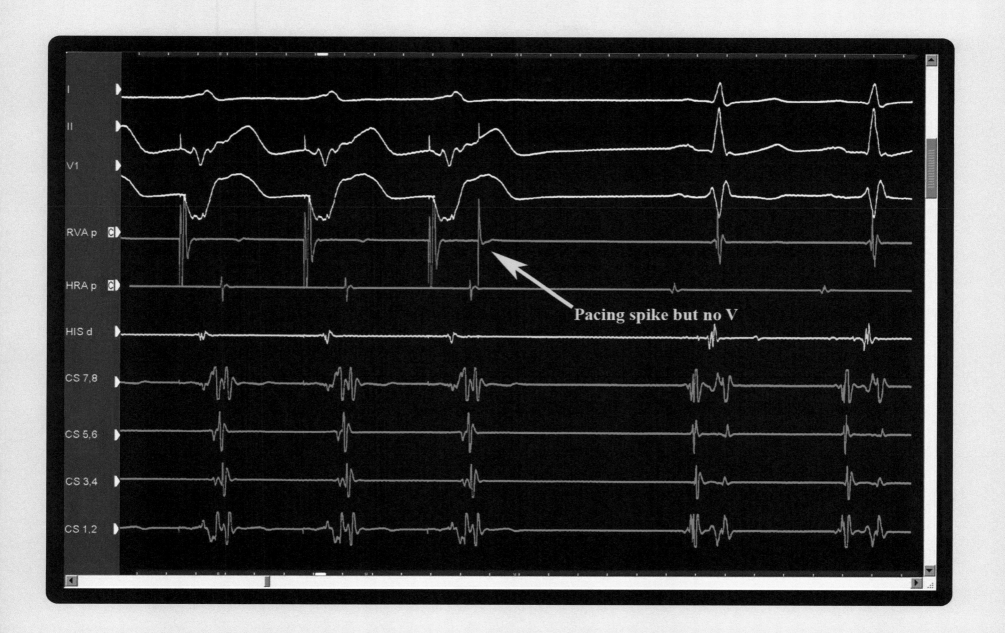

Pacing spike but no V

7. Supraventricular Tachycardia Diagnostic Study *continued*
Atrial Extra-stimulus Pacing

The next step in our diagnostic study is atrial extra-stimulus testing (S1-S2). This frequently induces our target tachycardia and allows us to evaluate the antegrade properties of the normal A-V conduction system (or AP if present). Since the AV node normally demonstrates decremental conduction, the A-H interval (*yellow arrows*) is a major focus of interest. Decremental conduction refers to the AV node's unique property of prolonging its conduction time in response to a shorter S1-S2 coupling interval. Hence, the A-H interval will become progressively longer as we shorten the S1-S2 coupling interval.

Note in this tracing that the A-H interval following the S2 is longer (*second arrow*) than the A-H interval during the S1 drive train (*first arrow*). An A-H interval typically begins at approximately 80 to 100 msec and lengthens (decrements) to slightly over 200 msec. An A-H interval longer than about 210 to 220 msec is often an indication that a second "slow" pathway is present. Typically, when a slow pathway is present, there is a sudden increase in the A-H interval as conduction blocks in the fast pathway and conducts more slowly over the slow pathway. This sudden increase in the A-H interval (>50 msec) with a 10-msec shortening of the S1-S2 coupling interval is often called a jump. See page 40.

Commentary: A jump reflects that we have reached the ERP of the fast pathway and conduction has shifted to a slower pathway. Absence of a jump does not preclude the presence of a slow pathway. A more sensitive way of discerning a jump is to plot a graph of A-H intervals against the S1-S2 coupling intervals to look for a more subtle discontinuity in the curve relating the A-H to prematurity of the extra-stimulus.

▶ Video 1.5: **Atrial Extra-stimulus Pacing**

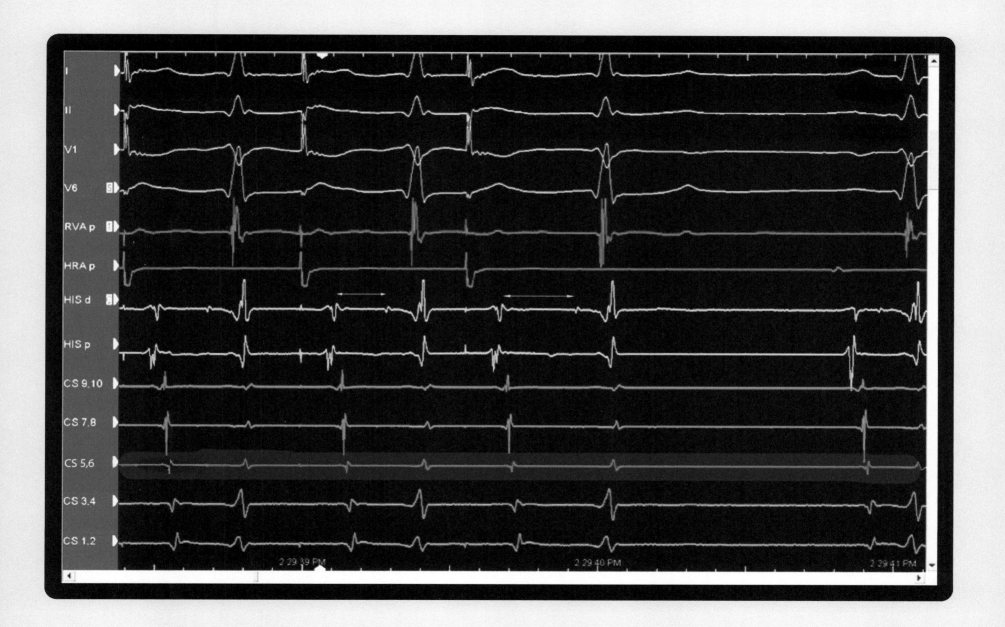

7. Supraventricular Tachycardia Diagnostic Study *continued*
Atrioventricular Block

As we continue to shorten the atrial S1-S2 coupling interval, we will eventually reach the antegrade ERP of the AV node, which is defined as the longest A1-A2 measured on the HIS channel that fails to conduct to the H. It is indicated on this tracing as a red atrial pacing spike (*arrow*) followed by evoked green CS A signals but no magenta V signal and no associated QRS on the surface ECG.

In a patient with dual AV nodal pathways, the situation is more complicated. In this example, both the slow pathway and the fast pathway ERPs have been reached.

Commentary: Once again, as we continue to shorten the S1-S2 coupling interval after achieving A-V block, we may observe unexpected return of conduction. See page 104 for more information about gap phenomenon.

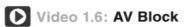 Video 1.6: **AV Block**

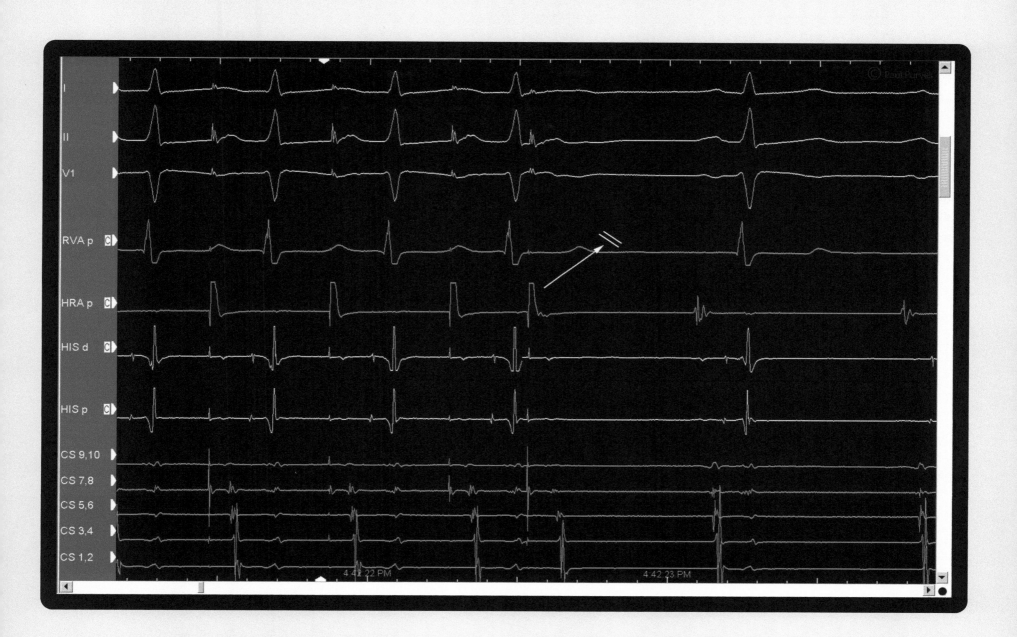

7. Supraventricular Tachycardia Diagnostic Study *continued*
Atrial Effective Refractory Period

Similar to what is discussed on page 26, as the S1-S2 coupling interval progressively shortens, we will reach the ERP of the atrial myocardium itself. Note on the drive train that each red spike is followed immediately by a yellow A on the HIS channels and a green A on the CS channels.

When myocardial ERP has been reached, the S2 does not generate an A signal on any channel.

We document this as NC. Remember again that this NC may be due to insufficient catheter contact. Repeat the drive to confirm NC.

Commentary: See the commentary on page 26. The same concepts apply in the atrium. Ensure good catheter placement, contact with the myocardium, sufficient current, and catheter stability throughout the study.

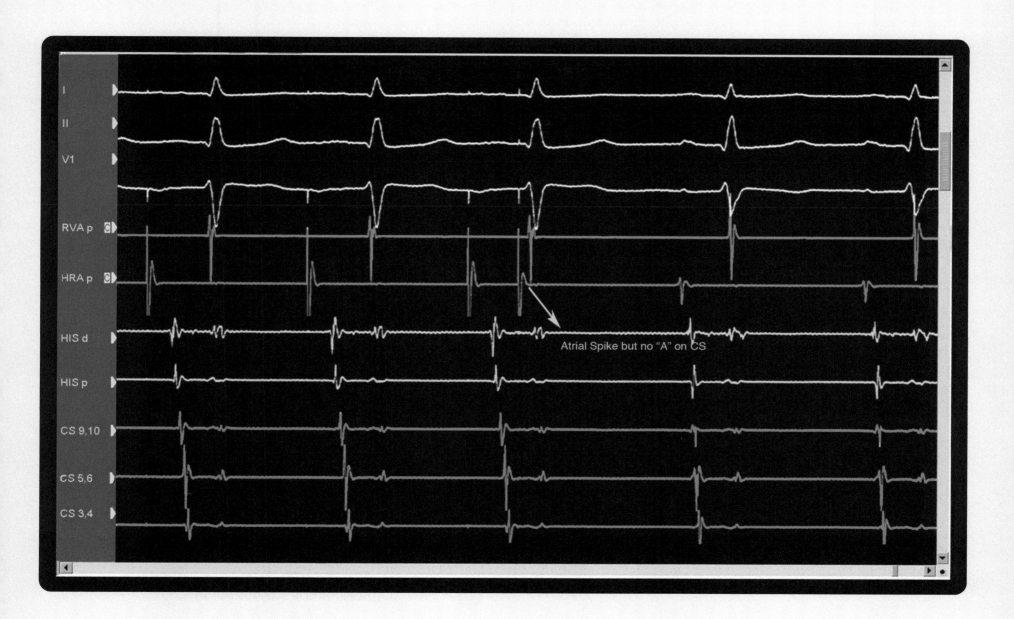

Atrial Spike but no "A" on CS

7. Supraventricular Tachycardia Diagnostic Study *continued*
Incremental Atrial Pacing

The final pacing maneuver in our routine diagnostic study is incremental atrial pacing. It establishes the antegrade block cycle length or antegrade Wenckebach point of the AV node. We do this last since incremental atrial pacing has the greatest potential to induce AF.

Note in this tracing that a red A pacing artifact is followed by a magenta VEGM in the RVA channel—until beat number 7. This atrial beat is not followed by a ventricular response. We therefore have reached the antegrade Wenckebach point of the AV node.

Also note that the AV node is decrementing (A-H is progressively increasing), as visualized by a longer distance between the A pace and the RVA response (*progressively longer arrows*). You can also see in the CS channels that the A-V distance is increasing.

Commentary: There are several points of interest here in addition to A-V block:

- Induction of a tachycardia
- A jump in the A-H interval during pacing
- Inadvertent induction of AF. Minimize the time that the pacing cycle length is less than 300 msec. Prolonged pacing at a rate of 250 msec or faster will often initiate AF. Be careful!

▶ Video 1.7: **Incremental Atrial Pacing**

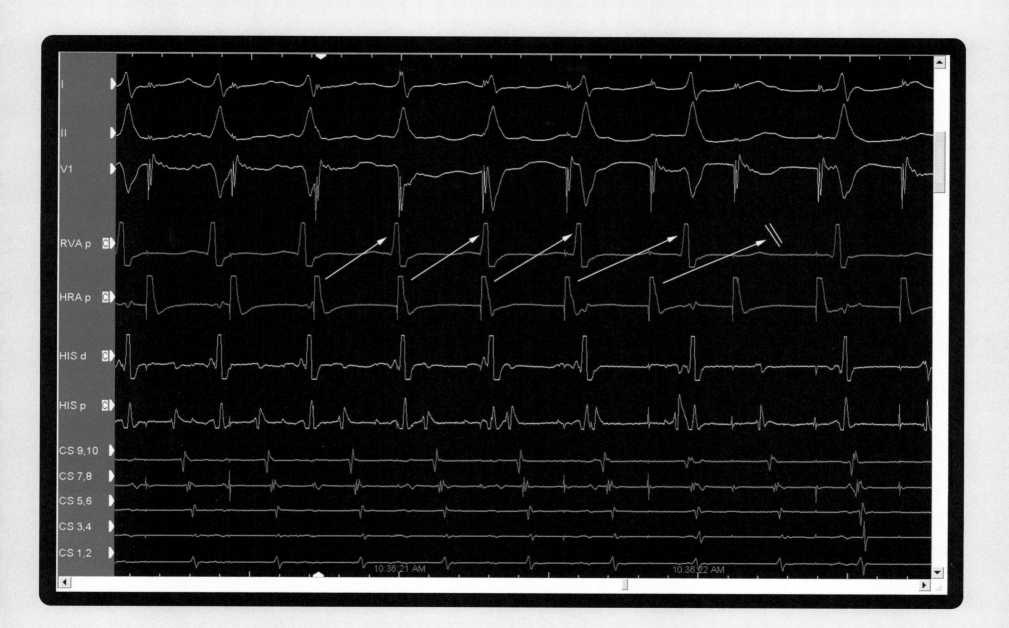

Unit 2:
Common Clinical Tachycardias

In this unit we examine the clinical mechanisms of the common tachycardias, which are well studied but incompletely understood. Perhaps it's better to say that our understanding of tachycardia mechanisms is under constant evolution.

Commentary: A key concept in this unit is reentry. Many, if not most, of the clinically important tachycardias are reentrant tachycardias, at least in part. The classic reentrant tachycardia requires two potential pathways of conduction that can be dissociated. These pathways are commonly thought of as a zone of fast conduction and a zone of slower conduction. The circuit is facilitated by this zone of slow conduction. Tachycardia is initiated by an ectopic beat that blocks in one zone and "reenters" via the other zone to initiate a "circus" or circular movement.

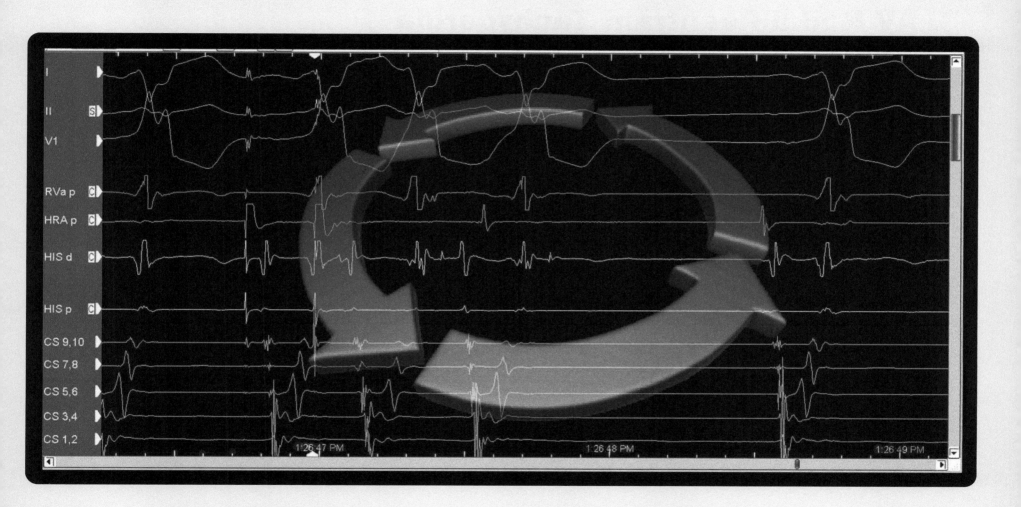

8. AV Nodal Reentrant Tachycardia
Typical AVNRT Pathways

AVNRT is possible in patients who have two routes over the AV node (dual AV nodal pathways). The exact anatomic substrate and location of these two pathways is not known with certainty, but it is undoubtedly true in theory and provides an excellent working concept.

Panel A shows a representation of the AV node with two routes through it, a fast pathway (F) and a slow pathway (S). This is known as longitudinal dissociation. During sinus rhythm, the wave of depolarization will travel quickly down the fast pathway to depolarize the ventricles. The same wave also travels down the slow pathway but finds the lower common pathway (LCP) refractory due to the preceding wavefront over the fast pathway.

Panel B introduces a premature atrial contraction (PAC) (S2) that blocks in the fast pathway due to the fast pathway's longer refractory period. Therefore, the S2 conducts to the ventricle using the slow pathway. Conduction using the slow pathway rather than the fast pathway means that there will be a sudden lengthening of the A-V interval (more specifically, lengthening of the A-H interval) or a jump.

As the wave of depolarization continues toward the ventricles, it also has the opportunity to travel retrogradely back up the fast pathway (*red arrows* in panels B and C) since the fast pathway has had sufficient time to recover.

This completes the circuit and initiates AVNRT, which is the continual "spinning" down the slow pathway and up the fast pathway.

Commentary: This is a good stylistic concept, but there are probably many mechanistic variants. For example, the diagram shows a common upper pathway entering the AV node when there is considerable evidence that there are two upper pathways entering the nodal area distinctively. An important practical point for ablation is that the slow pathway usually enters the AV node inferiorly near the CS orifice.

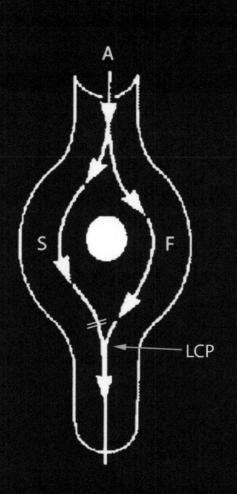
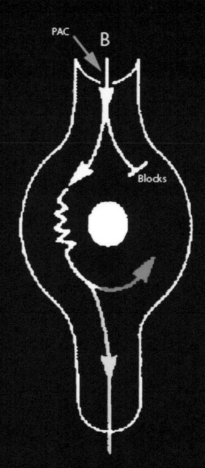
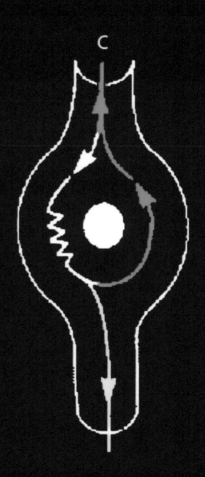

8. AV Nodal Reentrant Tachycardia *continued*
Jump

During sinus rhythm, in patients with dual AV nodal pathways, the two pathways are usually not apparent since fast pathway conduction preempts slow pathway conduction.

As you perform extra-stimulus testing (the S1-S2 extra-stimulus study), continue to measure the A-H interval generated by the S2. You will notice the A-H interval gradually lengthening as the fast AV nodal pathway decrements. A sudden, abrupt prolongation of the A-H interval signals a block in the fast pathway and transition to the slow pathway (*arrows*). This jump is an indication that we have reached the ERP of the fast pathway and conduction to the ventricles is now occurring via the slow pathway. By arbitrary definition we consider at least a 50-msec prolongation in the A-H interval with a 10-msec shortening of the S1-S2 coupling interval to be a significant jump.

This dual AV nodal physiology is the substrate for AVNRT. Generally, slow pathways are associated with A-H intervals ranging from 250 to 700 msec or longer.

Commentary: Dual AV nodal pathways may exist without AVNRT, and AVNRT may exist without apparent dual pathways. In addition, AVNRT may be quite difficult to initiate. Using two extra-stimuli (S2-S3) or more and pacing at multiple sites may help. Isoproterenol or atropine may facilitate induction as well.

▶ Video 2.1: **Slow Pathway**

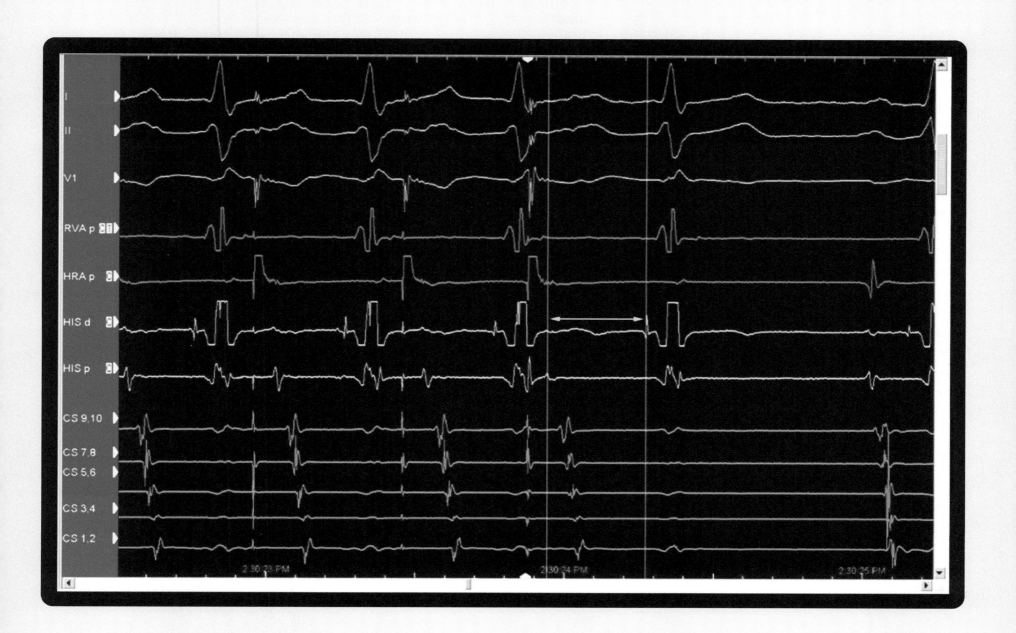

8. AV Nodal Reentrant Tachycardia *continued*
AV Nodal Echo

Before any tachycardia is induced, we often see an AV nodal "echo" (*white arrows*). An echo is defined as a beat that returns to its origin (back to the atrium from the paced atrial cycle in this context) and is, in actuality, a single beat of reentrant tachycardia.

In this example, we are pacing the right atrium. The first three beats (S1) are paced at a constant interval followed by an S2. We can see that each atrial pacing artifact is associated with atrial capture and subsequent conduction to the ventricle. However, on the fourth paced beat (S2), following conduction to the ventricle, we see another AEGM. In other words, we paced the A, which led to the expected V, and then an extra, unexpected A returned to the atrium. Hence, the term "echo beat." This can be thought of as one beat of AVNRT.

Commentary: Notice the A-H interval is relatively short and constant for the first three paced beats. On the fourth paced beat, notice that the A-H interval is much longer. This indicates that conduction has blocked in the antegrade fast AV nodal pathway and now is conducting over a slower AV nodal pathway. This is followed by retrograde conduction back to the atrium (echo beat). There is subsequent conduction block antegradely in the slow pathway (otherwise sustained AVNRT would have been initiated).

▶ Video 2.2: **AV Nodal Echo**

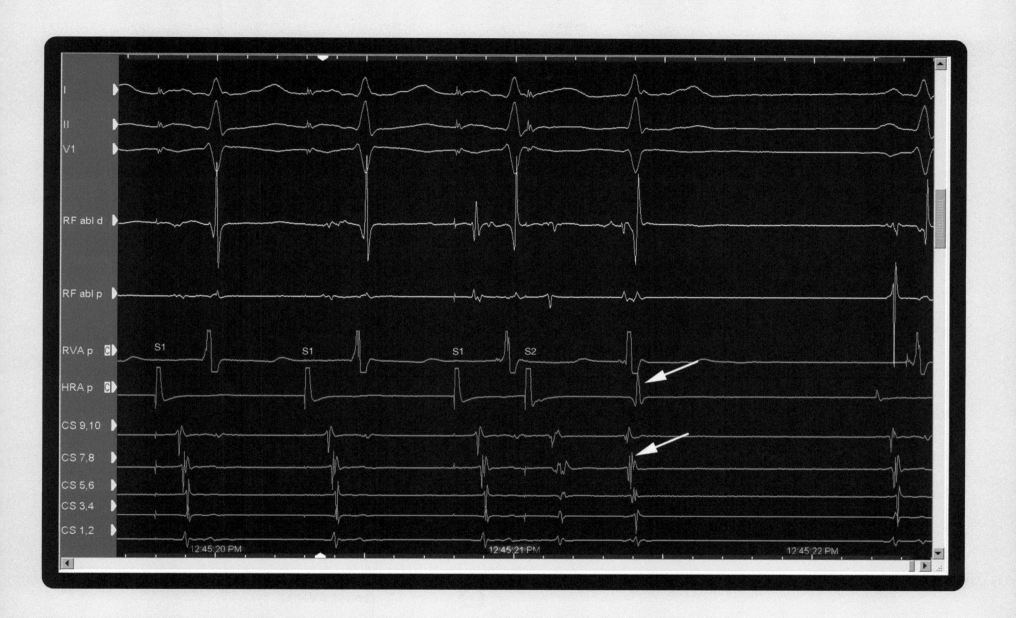

8. AV Nodal Reentrant Tachycardia *continued*
Onset of Tachycardia

This image shows the typical onset of AVNRT. Note of the length of the A-H interval on the HIS channel during the drive train. Focus on the S2 (the last red paced beat immediately under the magenta V). It generates the green A signals on the CS channels. We then see a rather lengthy flat line. This represents the transit time through the AV node via the slow pathway (*long yellow arrow*). When the wave of depolarization finally exits the AV node, the yellow HIS channel displays an H signal followed by a large yellow V signal.

While the wave of depolarization is traveling from the HIS channel to the ventricle (*short white arrow*), it also travels back up to the right atrium via a retrograde fast pathway (*short red arrow*), thus generating the red A that can be seen immediately under the magenta V. If this happens once or twice, we call these cycles "AV nodal echo beats." If these cycles continue, we have initiated AVNRT. In this example, we can see two echo beats.

Because this particular reentrant circuit allows conduction antegradely down the slow AV nodal pathway and retrogradely up the fast pathway, it is often referred to as "slow-fast" or "typical" AVNRT. It is the most common form of AV nodal reentry seen clinically.

The S1-S2 coupling interval blocks in the fast pathway (antegrade ERP of the AV nodal fast pathway) and continues over the slow pathway. Tachycardia is cured with successful ablation of the slow pathway, which is an obligatory link in the circuit.

Commentary: Ablating a slow pathway must be done with great care due to its close proximity to the AV node. If the patient suddenly takes a deep breath or moves during ablation, the catheter may "ride up" toward the AV node, potentially causing temporary or permanent complete AV block.

▶ Video 2.3: **Onset AVNRT**

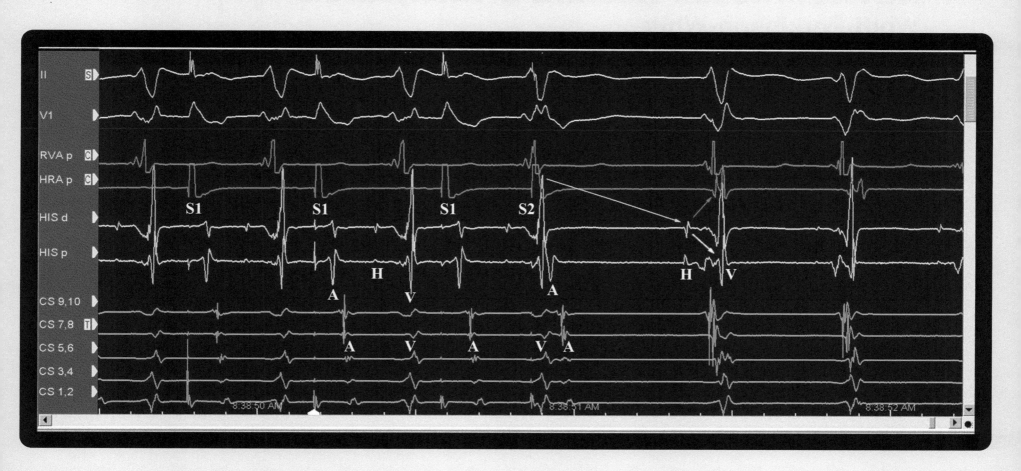

9. Atrioventricular Reentrant Tachycardia
Wolff-Parkinson-White

Wolff, Parkinson, and White are the three physicians who first described a syndrome in a group of patients who showed a widened, slurred QRS complex and suffered from recurrent bouts of tachycardia. WPW *syndrome* refers to patients who have pre-excitation *and* suffer from tachycardias. Patients who display ventricular pre-excitation on the ECG but don't have tachycardias are said to have a WPW *pattern*.

In the normal individual, the only electrical connection between the atria and ventricles is the AV node. APs are electrically conducting myocardial tissues that bridge the atria and ventricles in addition to the normal AV node. When this connection conducts electrical activity from the atria to the ventricles earlier than expected (pre-excitation), it manifests on the surface ECG as a widened, slurred QRS. This "delta wave" refers to the initial part of this widened QRS that represents conduction directly into the ventricle.

Some APs cannot conduct electrical activity from the atria to the ventricles (antegrade conduction). They can only conduct from the ventricles to the atria (retrograde conduction). If the pathway conducts retrogradely only, there will be no pre-excitation on the ECG even though the AP is present (see lower panel). This is not WPW (by classic definition), but these APs still can cause reentrant tachycardia by virtue of their retrograde conduction alone.

Commentary: In AVNRT, the reentry occurs over two pathways in close proximity to the AV node itself. With APs, another pathway is present in addition to the AV node allowing A-V reentry. Typically, the reentrant circuit is "down" the AV node and "up" the AP. The circuit can also go down the AP and back up the AV node. If more than one AP is present, the possibility of a "pathway to pathway" reentrant tachycardia exists.

▶ Video 2.4: **Left Lateral AP**

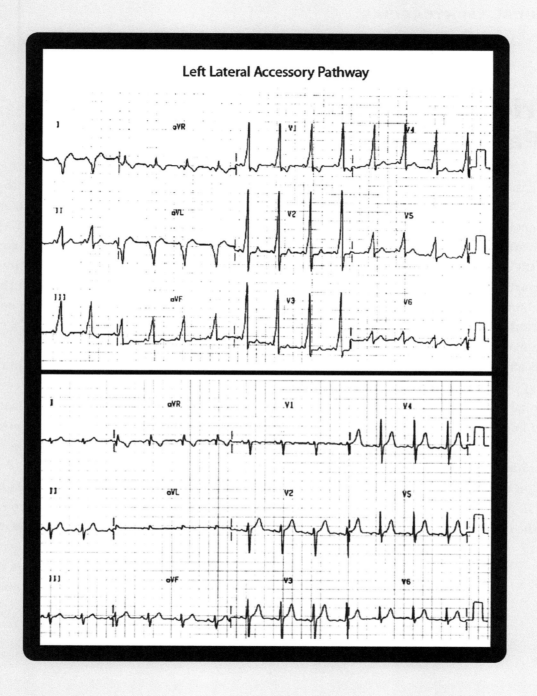

Left Lateral Accessory Pathway

9. Atrioventricular Reentrant Tachycardia *continued*
Accessory Pathway Locations

APs can occur anywhere along the AV rings: They may be right-sided, left-sided, peri-nodal, or septal. They can conduct antegradely only, retrogradely only or, more commonly, bidirectionally. In an antegradely conducting AP, the atrial activation wavefront has two routes to the ventricles, the AV node and the AP. If the atrial impulse conducts over the AP to depolarize a part of the ventricular myocardium in advance of the AV nodal–His bundle depolarization wavefront, then the AP is "pre-exciting" the ventricles; hence the term "ventricular pre-excitation" or simply "pre-excitation." Ventricular pre-excitation appears on the surface ECG as an initial slurring of the QRS upstroke or delta wave. Delta waves may be subtle or obvious, depending on a number of factors that determine how much of ventricular activation is due to the AP versus the AV node.

If a pathway conducts retrogradely only, we consider it "concealed" since there is no pre-excitation on the ECG and the spresence of a pathway is not apparent. This implies that the only way the AP can be involved in a tachycardia is if the reentrant circuit involves conduction from the atrium, down the AV node to the ventricles, and back up to the atria using the AP (generating a narrow QRS tachycardia). This mechanism is called "orthodromic" AVRT. If the pathway conducts antegradely only, the ECG will show various degrees of pre-excitation. These pathways can only become involved in "antidromic" AVRT, meaning that the circuit goes from the atrium, down the AP to the ventricles, and back up to the atria using the AV node (generating a wide QRS tachycardia).

Most pathways exhibit bidirectional conduction properties and therefore will exhibit various degrees of pre-excitation; thus tachycardia can potentially be orthodromic or antidromic. Orthodromic tachycardia is much more common.

Commentary: Five percent of patients have more than one AP. A tachycardia could potentially go from pathway to pathway and not involve the AV node at all. This would mean that the circuit goes from the atrium, down to the ventricles using one AP, and back up to the atria using a second AP. This is an uncommon tachycardia and demonstrates a wide QRS morphology.

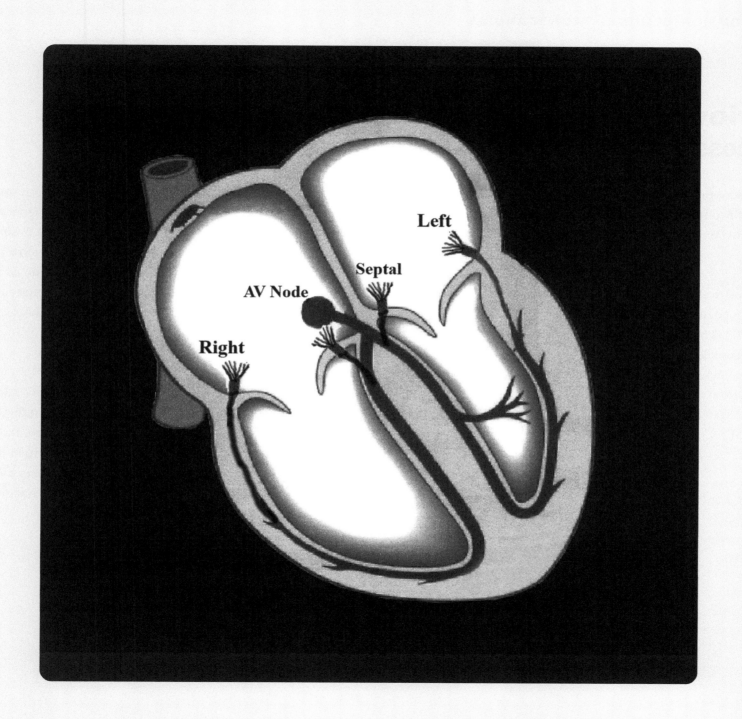

9. Atrioventricular Reentrant Tachycardia *continued*
Accessory Pathway Echo

When delivering programmed extra-stimuli, we often see a single echo beat prior to initiating tachycardia. Recall that an echo beat is essentially one beat of reentrant tachycardia (see page 42 to review echo beats).

In this example, we are pacing in the ventricle. Notice how the atrial activation is eccentric, indicating a left lateral AP (CS 1-2 is the earliest AEGM). The S2 continues to be conducted to the atrium via the AP as diagnosed by the early atrial signal in CS 1-2.

After the AEGM (on the HIS channel), we then see a long A-H interval (*yellow arrow*) followed by a VEGM. This indicates that after conduction to the atrium using the AP, there is conduction back over the AV node to the ventricle, likely using a slow pathway. This is a single echo beat using the AP and the AV node as the circuit. In fact, there is conduction back to the atrium one more time using the AP (*white arrows*). So we really have one and a half cycles of AVRT before it stops by blocking in the AV node.

Commentary: Why did the AP echo not initiate AVRT? To answer this, we simply need to consider what the weak link is in this reentrant circuit. The last activity was an AEGM received from the AP. The tachycardia was prevented because of blocking in the AV node. This makes the AV node the "weak link." Starting the patient on isoproterenol to improve AV nodal conduction may allow AVRT initiation.

▶ Video 2.5: **AP Echos**

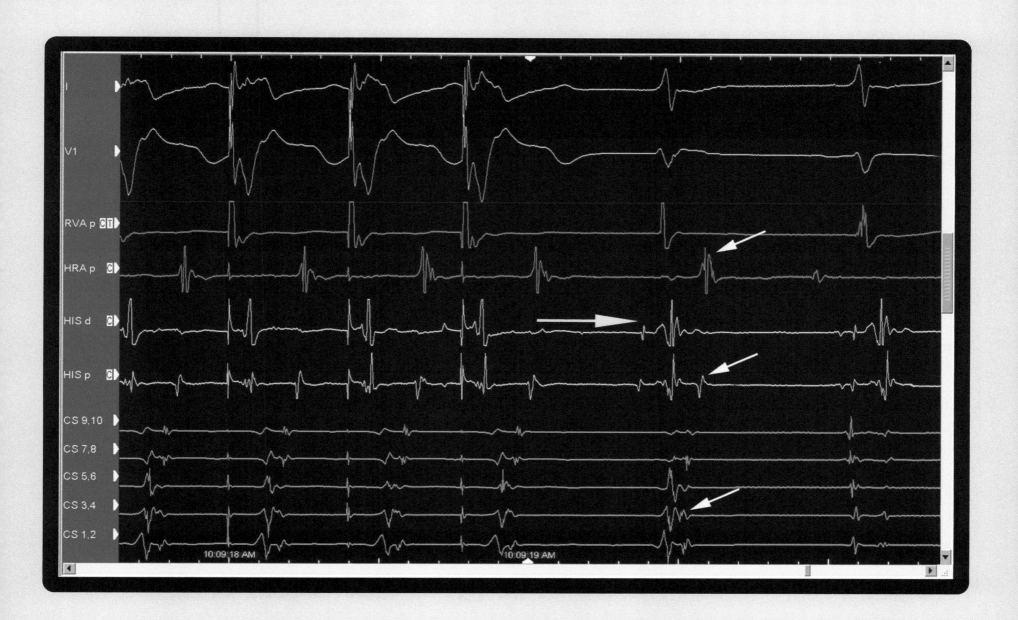

9. Atrioventricular Reentrant Tachycardia *continued*
AVRT Initiation

This is a typical onset of AVRT. Recall the really slow pathway that initiated AVNRT on page 44. On this tracing there is a similar slow pathway over the AV node (see the A-H interval on the HIS channel and the *yellow arrow*). However, in this example, there is no retrograde fast pathway up the AV node. Instead, there is retrograde conduction via a left lateral AP to the left atrium (*green arrow*). If we examine the CS activation, we see that CS 1-2 has the first A, followed by CS 3-4, CS 5-6, CS 7-8, then the HIS A, and finally the HRA A. This atrial activation sequence is known as eccentric atrial activation. The AP joins the atrium and ventricle in the vicinity of CS 1-2, and hence the atria are activated from the left atrium to the right atrium. This is, of course, the exact opposite of normal atrial activation.

All reentrant tachycardia circuits require a zone of relatively slow conduction. In AVRT, this zone is generally the AV node and the alternate pathway is the AP.

Therefore, in the common orthodromic AVRT, the circuit is from the atrium, down the node (*yellow arrow*) to the ventricle, and back to the atrium via the AP (*green arrow*). The tachycardia then continues. The usual cure is to ablate the AP. With your most common approach (transseptal or retrograde aortic), an ablation catheter will be advanced into the left atrium and placed directly on the pathway. Radiofrequency energy is applied and the pathway is eliminated. In this example, the pathway is in the lateral left atrium as suggested by the earliest atrial signal in CS 1-2.

Commentary: You may also notice that all the QRS complexes are not pre-excited. This patient clearly has no antegrade conduction over the AP or, at this pacing cycle length, the ERP of the AP has been reached.

▶ Video 2.6: **AVRT Initiation**

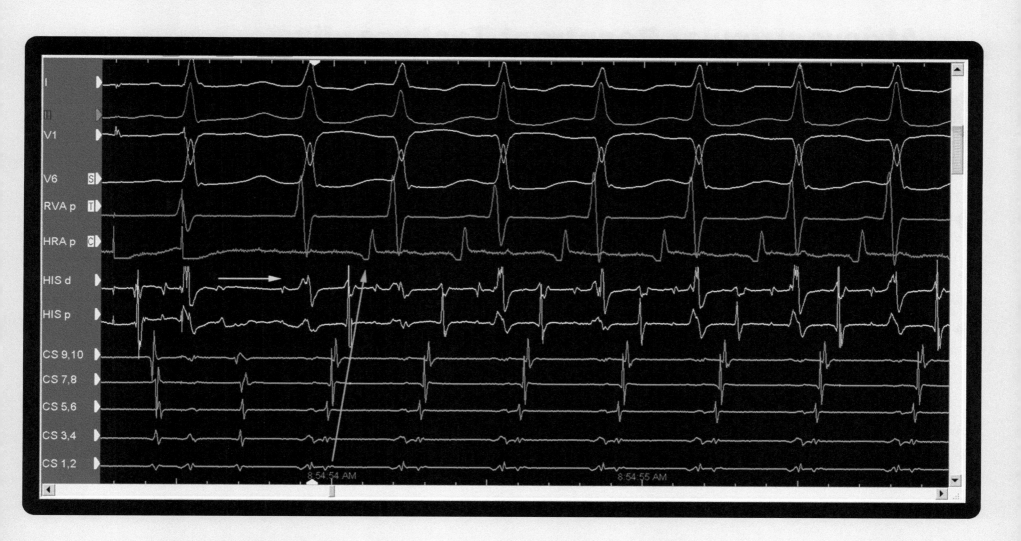

9. Atrioventricular Reentrant Tachycardia *continued*
AVRT Initiation

In this tracing, similar to the previous tracing, a left lateral AP is revealed and tachycardia initiated. But how? Where is the zone of slow conduction?

The required conduction delay when AVRT is initiated (by an S2) is provided by a delay in the A-H interval in most instances. Initiation of this tachycardia is unique in that it is a long H-V interval (*white arrows*) that provides the required conduction delay.

Commentary: H-V interval prolongation is due to a slowing of conduction in the His-Purkinje system. Decrement in the His-Purkinje system can be observed normally after a "long–short" sequence; that is, the stimulation results in a long cycle (the last S1-S1) followed by a short cycle (S1-S2), especially if the A-H interval is very short as in this individual. A more detailed explanation of this phenomenon can be found in other textbooks.

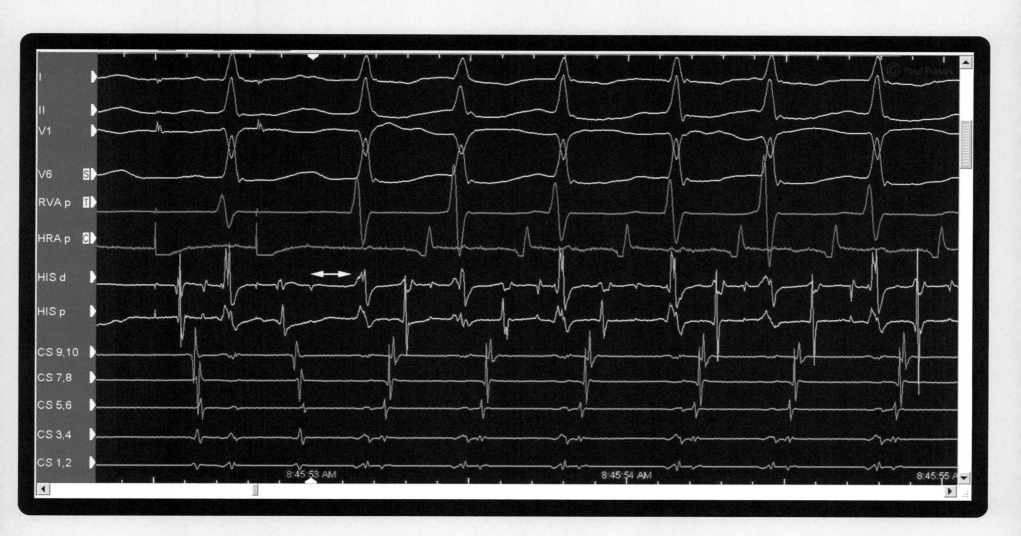

9. Atrioventricular Reentrant Tachycardia *continued*
AVRT Initiation

In this example, the AVRT is initiated by quite a different mechanism. The S2 from the HRA is conducted to the ventricles, but the surface ECG shows that the QRS complex has a left bundle branch block (LBBB) pattern.

Normally, the ventricular activation would get to the left-sided AP via the left bundle branch. Since the S2 was given at a time when the left bundle branch system was refractory (thus the LBBB pattern), the wave of depolarization had to get there via the right bundle, then transseptally to the left ventricle and finally to the left lateral AP.

Propagation of the impulse through muscle is not as rapid as over the normal conduction system, hence the impulse gets to the AP much later than expected. The AP is now recovered fully due to this delay and is able to propagate to the atrium and initiate tachycardia.

Commentary: This only occurs when the AP is on the same side (ipsilateral) as the bundle branch block. With a right-sided AP, a RBBB would facilitate initiation of tachycardia. The wave of depolarization would travel down the left bundle, then transseptally to the right ventricle and up the right-sided pathway. So the next logical question would be, "Would an RBBB cause initiation of AVRT that uses a left lateral AP?" The answer is no. A contralateral bundle branch block will not facilitate initiation of tachycardia since that bundle is not part of the circuit.

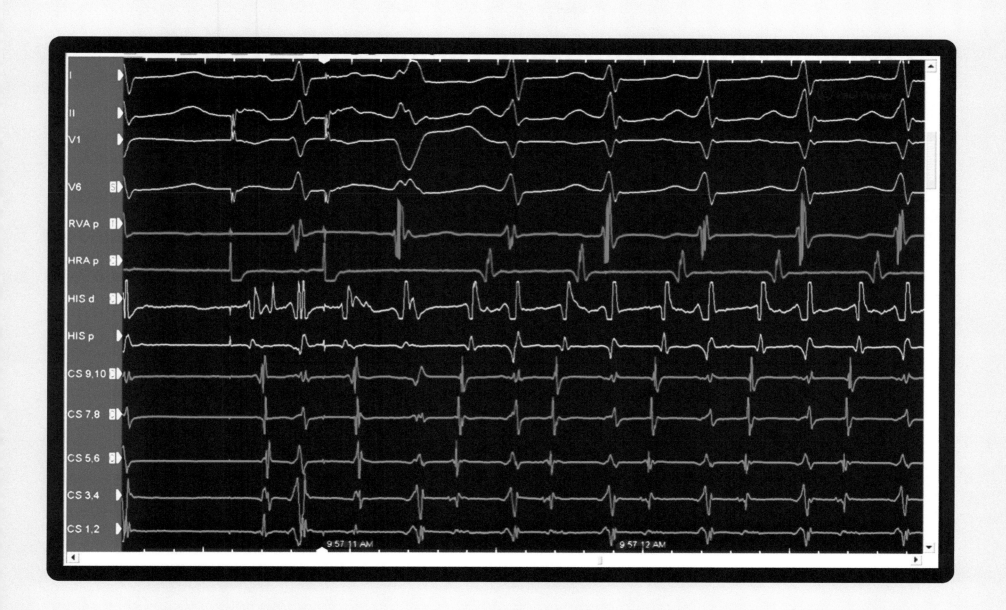

9. Atrioventricular Reentrant Tachycardia *continued*
Effective Refractory Period of an Accessory Pathway

During the atrial drive (S1), the QRS complex shows pre-excitation (WPW pattern). It is a left lateral AP since lead I is mostly negative and V1 shows an RBBB-like pattern.

Notice that during the atrial drive train the QRS is markedly pre-excited with no contribution of ventricular activation from the normal conduction system. This "maximum pre-excitation" is due to the wave of depolarization reaching the left lateral AP earlier than the AV node, which obviously must have a long conduction time.

After the S2, the A-H interval (*yellow arrow*) is very long and the QRS is no longer pre-excited. At this S1-S2 coupling interval, the antegrade ERP of the AP has been reached, allowing conduction exclusively over the AV node over a slow pathway, thus displaying a long A-H interval.

After traveling over the AV node via a slow pathway, the wave of depolarization then "echoes" back up to the left atrium via the left lateral AP (*green arrow*). This might initiate ongoing AVRT, but in this example we have only a single AP echo.

Commentary: The weak limb of the circuit at this particular moment is the AV node. Administration of atropine or isoproterenol may facilitate induction of sustained tachycardia.

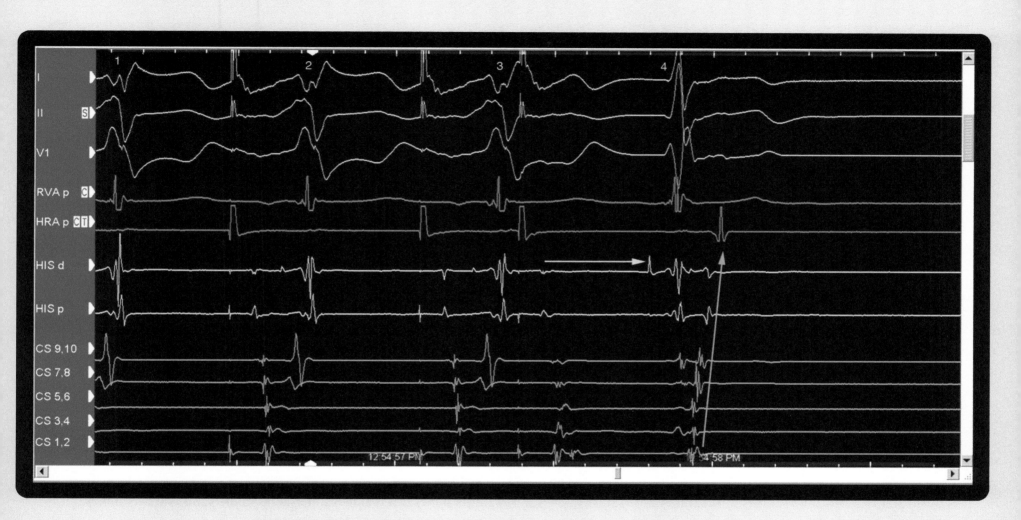

9. Atrioventricular Reentrant Tachycardia *continued*
Ablation of Accessory Pathways

The overall principle of AP localization is quite simple. When the AP is being used to activate either the atrium or the ventricle, the part of that chamber that is activated first will identify the location of the AP. During ventricular pacing (as in this example), we are moving our mapping or ablation catheter looking for the earliest atrial activation. Similarly, during atrial pacing, we would be looking for the earliest ventricular activation.

The concept is more easily clarified by this diagram, which illustrates the morphology of the EGMs during ventricular pacing. Therefore, the earliest atrial signal should identify where the AP inserts into the left atrium.

In the left panel, we move the catheter to a location where we believe the AP inserts into the atrium. The ablation channels show the V and A signals on both the distal and proximal poles. Notice that the signals are separated by several milliseconds. At this point in the mapping sequence, we don't know whether this is the earliest and will not know until we have finished mapping, but the separation of the V and A signals suggests we can do better.

In the right panel, we have moved the catheter to a slightly different location. Notice now that the A signal is much earlier and that the VEGM and AEGM are fused together and frankly overlapping. This looks to be a promising ablation site perhaps directly over the AP, but this is only established by careful mapping of the region.

Commentary: Notice as well in the left panel that the AEGM is biphasic with an initial "shoulder" of far-field activity prior to the rapid downslope indicating local activation. This also suggests that this is not an ideal ablation site. The A is so early on the right panel that it actually merges with the V, so one can't really comment on the AEGM morphology.

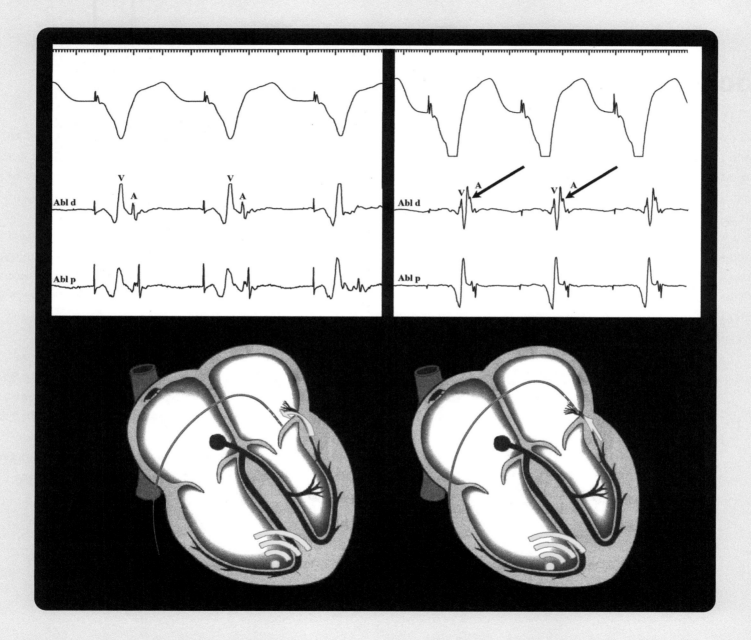

10. Focal Atrial Tachycardia

Focal atrial tachycardias originate from a small area or point source in either atrium (*pink star*). They are not as common as WPW or AVNRT and are often more challenging to ablate. The first challenge is to reproducibly initiate the tachycardia in the lab. Unlike a slow pathway ablation, which has a known anatomic target or an AP that can be localized without initiating tachycardia, atrial tachycardia can only be localized and targeted for ablation during ongoing tachycardia. The mechanism of initiation is variable (automaticity versus triggered versus micro-reentry) and often difficult to determine, but the key clinical consideration is whether it is present during the study or can be induced by programmed stimulation or isoproterenol.

Once initiated, detailed activation mapping is the necessary prerequisite to successful ablation. This involves determining the atrial activation sequence and finding the earliest atrial signal during the tachycardia (similar to WPW).

An activation sequence map is obtained with an electroanatomic mapping system. It is very useful and frequently employed with focal AT. Pace mapping and entrainment mapping are additional techniques that may be helpful, but the whole ablation exercise is very difficult without activation mapping.

Commentary: So how do we know that we are not simply entraining sinus tachycardia? If we have an ectopic focus and entrain quite close to it, the post-pacing interval (PPI)–tachycardia cycle length (TCL) may be 20 msec or less. If it's the SA node, the PPI–TCL never gets smaller than approximately 80 msec. The SA node seems to be "protected" and thus we can't get closer than 80 msec.

Video 2.7: **Focal Atrial Tachycardia**

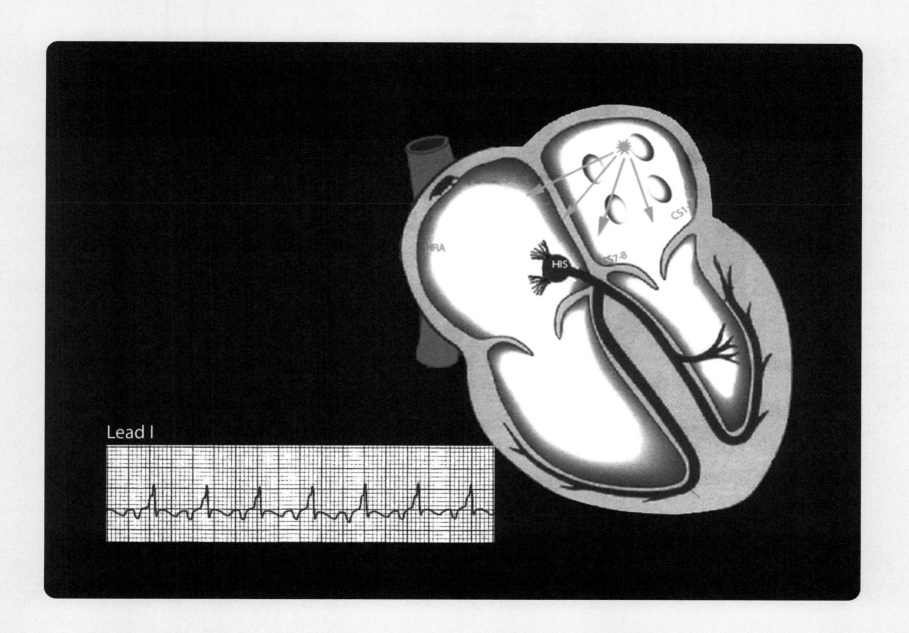

Lead I

11. Atrial Flutter
Typical Catheter Placement

Atrial flutter is a specific atrial tachycardia characterized by an atrial rate in range of 250 bpm. In the great majority of patients, atrial flutter is related to a large reentrant circuit in the right atrium that has to pass through a relatively small area, namely the narrow band of muscle between the inferior vena cava and the tricuspid valve known as the CTI.

This image shows a commonly seen placement of catheters for CTI-dependent atrial flutter ablation. The *red arrows* point to a duo-decapolar ("duo-deca") catheter positioned around the right atrium, anterior to the crista terminalis. The *white arrow* points to the ablation catheter positioned at the CTI. The *magenta arrow* indicates the RVA catheter for ventricular pacing if needed. The *green arrows* point to a CS catheter for atrial pacing. The arrow colors correspond to the colors of the EGMs on our monitor.

The CTI in this projection (*dotted yellow line*) is positioned so that the distal electrode pair is at the ventricular part of the "isthmus" near the tricuspid valve ring. The catheter would have to be withdrawn to cover the isthmus and reach the inferior vena cava end. The line of ablation will proceed along this curved yellow line.

Commentary: Catheter placement is again important. The duo-deca catheter should ideally be placed anterior to the crista terminalis to obtain useful mapping of the direction of activation. For proper signal interpretation, the catheter operator needs to establish this using multi-plane fluoroscopy or a mapping system.

▶ Video 2.8: **Typical CCW CTI-dependent Atrial Flutter**

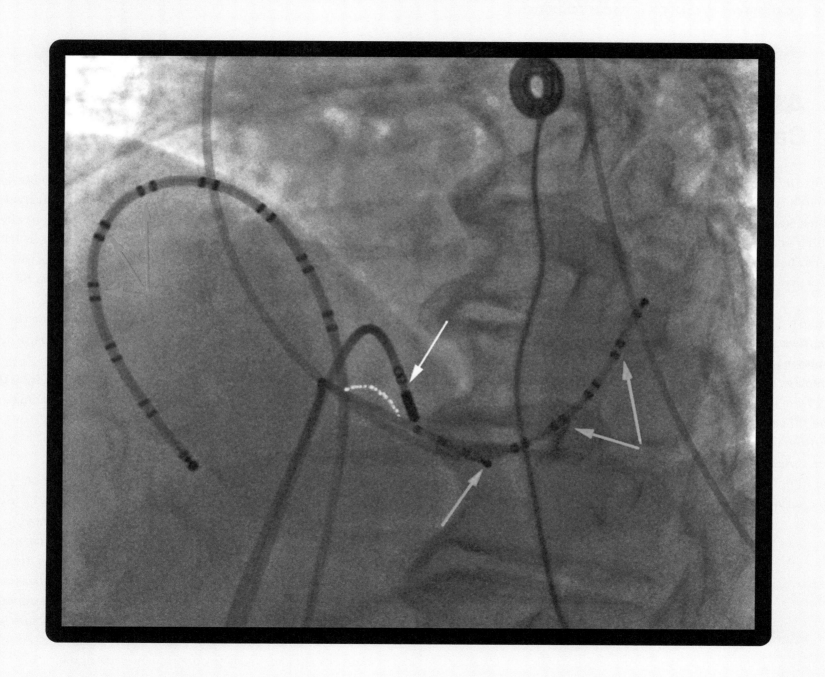

11. **Atrial Flutter** *continued*
Cavo-tricuspid Isthmus Ablation

In this example, the patient arrived in sinus rhythm but has had documented typical atrial flutter clinically. The ablation strategy will be to block conduction over the CTI to prevent tachycardia. There is no compelling need to induce the tachycardia in the laboratory if we are confident about the diagnosis from the clinical ECGs, although some clinicians may choose to induce atrial flutter and verify the mechanism.

To evaluate CTI conduction, it is helpful to pace at one end of the isthmus. We start by pacing the proximal CS (CS 7-8). The red channels are displaying a 20-pole duo-deca catheter. In the left panel, the duo-deca displays a chevron shape (*arrows*). The wave of depolarization spreads from the CS os toward the right atrial lateral wall inferiorly over the CTI (starting at low right atrial [LRA] catheter 1-2) and superiorly up the atrial septum (starting at HRA 17-18). The wavefronts meet somewhere in the atrium in the vicinity of mid right atrial (MRA) catheter 9-10. This double-wavefront pattern is characteristic of intact CTI conduction.

After successful ablation (right panel), the chevron or double-wavefront shape is replaced with a straight single-wavefront activation line (*arrow*). The sequence of activation shows the wavefront circulating counter-clockwise around the right atrium beginning at HRA 17-18 with LRA 1-2 last. This would be expected if the isthmus were blocked in the clockwise direction, allowing the right atrium to be activated only up the septum. Note also that LRA 1-2, LRA 3-4, and LRA 5-6 EGM polarity has reversed. This is further proof that the wave of depolarization has arrived at these poles from the opposite direction.

Finally, we will pace from LRA 1-2 to observe CTI block from the other direction. CS pacing confirms clockwise block. LRA pacing confirms counterclockwise block. Bidirectional block is critical!

Commentary: If the duo-deca catheter is positioned properly with poles 1-2 in the lateral LRA relatively close to the CTI, the CS to LRA time with an intact CTI is approximately 80 msec. The LRA to CS os time is similar. When CTI block is achieved, these times generally will double since conduction from the CS to LRA is no longer directly over the CTI but goes circumferentially around the right atrium. It is important to note that slow conduction through the CTI can be present and mimic total block. There is no absolute number that is diagnostic of CTI block. Other maneuvers are necessary to confirm complete block.

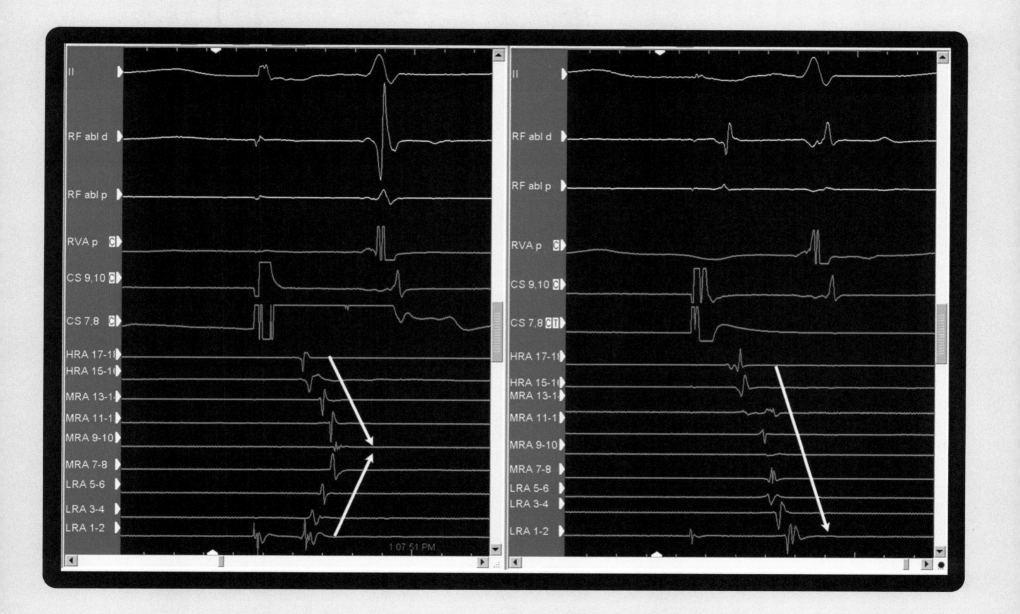

11. **Atrial Flutter** *continued*
Split A's

A "split" A refers to an AEGM with two apparent depolarizations or components. The recording electrodes of an ablation catheter cover a relatively large area so that it is possible to record depolarizations from more than one region in that area. Seeing an early and a later A in this context suggests two waves of depolarization, one on each side of the ablation line. The early component represents atrial activation on one side of the line, and the late component represents the delayed activation as it arrives at the other side of the line. As the ablation proceeds and tissue along the CTI is damaged, the split may appear due to slower, injury-related conduction. The split will lengthen during ablation, sometimes abruptly but often gradually, until total block is achieved. The late A arrives by an entirely different route (by going around the right atrium rather than over the blocked isthmus). In general, atrial conduction time around the right atrium, in either direction, is at least 80 msec so that a split of less than 80 msec suggests that the CTI is not blocked. The wider the split, the more likely that block is present; but no absolute number is entirely reliable to distinguish complete block from slow isthmus conduction. Other maneuvers are necessary.

Notice on the distal ablation channel, after the CS pacing spike on beats 1 and 2, there are two narrowly split A-waves with a split of 40 msec (*shorter red arrows*). On beats 3 and 4, the A-waves have split further (140 msec; *longer red arrows*). This occurred during ablation.

Commentary: Distinguishing slow conduction over the CTI from total block can be difficult. A maneuver sometimes called "differential pacing" may be helpful. Simply pacing at a site closer to the line will delay arrival at the other side (widen the split) if complete block is present, while it will do the opposite if in fact conduction is still occurring, albeit slowly, over the CTI.

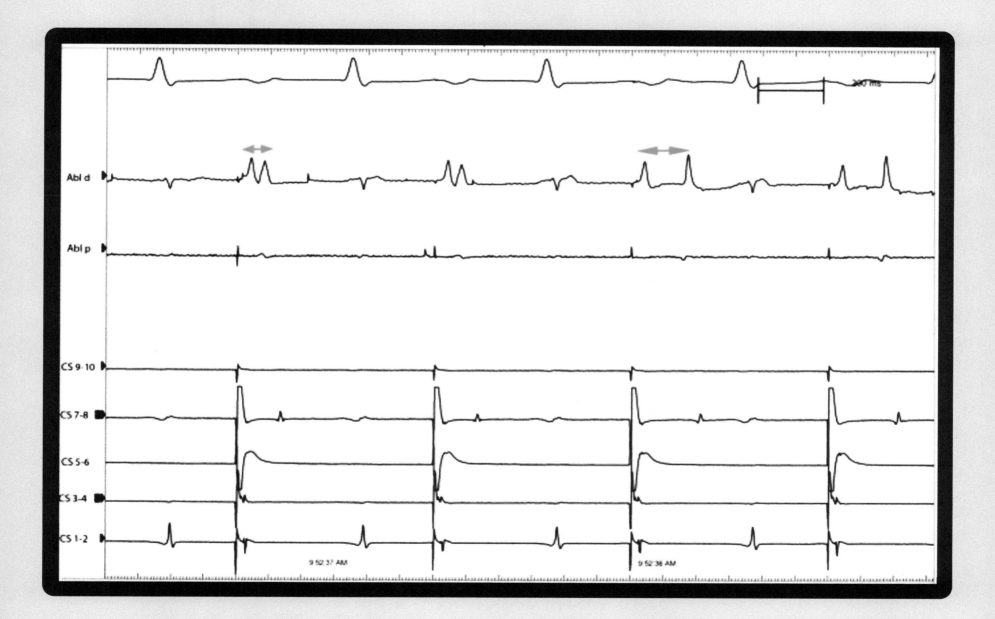

12. Atrial Fibrillation
Basic Diagnosis

AF entails disorganized electrical activity throughout the atria, typically causing palpitations and lasting hours (paroxysmal), days, or longer (persistent). Unlike atrial flutter, AVNRT, AVRT, or atrial tachycardia, AF is disorganized atrial activity involving the entire left and right atria and there is no simple target for ablation. However, we now know that AF usually requires a trigger to start it and sufficient substrate to maintain it. Therefore, we attempt to reduce the frequency of AF episodes by eliminating the most common triggers that arise from the four pulmonary veins (PVs) in the back of the left atrium.

Our goal for ablation, therefore, is to electrically isolate the PVs so that ectopy from the veins does not enter the left atrium and cause AF. In this image, we have positioned a lasso-shaped duo-decapolar catheter (Lasso™ Circular Mapping Catheter, Biosense Webster, Diamond Bar, California, USA; *green arrow*) in the left inferior PV. The *yellow arrow* points to the ablation catheter, the *magenta arrow* points to the CS catheter, and the *black arrow* points to an esophageal temperature probe.

In this example, we will pace from CS 1-2 and observe the wave of depolarization traveling into the left inferior PV. With ablation around the veins, the EGMs recorded on the Lasso catheter will disappear once we have achieved PV entrance block. To test for exit block, we pace one or more of the poles on the Lasso and observe whether conduction reaches the left atrium. Exit block is defined as local capture within the PV while observing that it does not exit into the left atrium and thus generate a P-wave on the surface ECG.

Commentary: PV entrance block can be observed occasionally while conduction remains intact from vein to atrium (ie, lack of exit block). It seems intuitive that exit block is the more important goal since ectopy in the veins exits to initiate AF. Therefore, most labs target bidirectional block, although there can be technical challenges in achieving capture in the vein in some patients.

▶ Video 2.9: **Atrial Fibrillation**

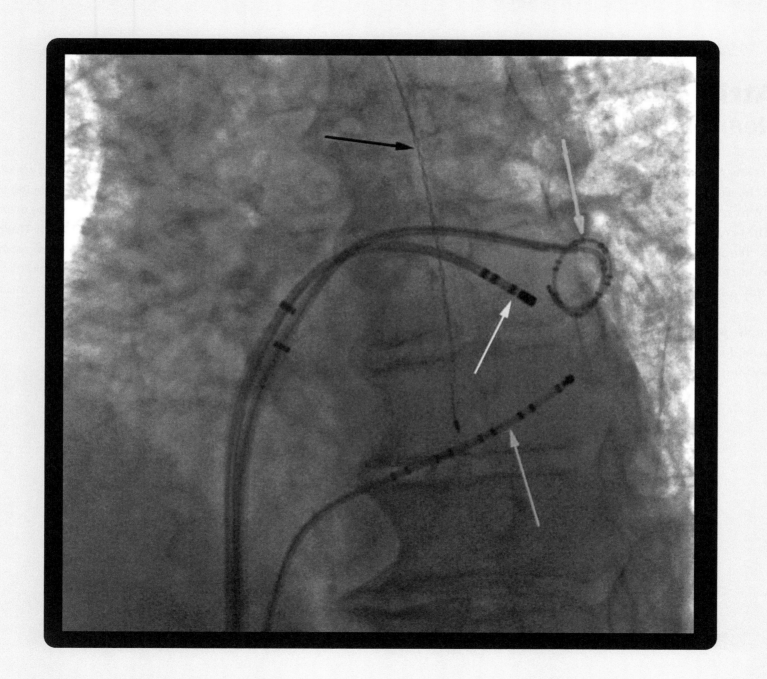

12. **Atrial Fibrillation** *continued*
Near-Field Versus Far-Field Electrograms

It is important to appreciate the different morphologies of EGMs and the relationship with distance from the recording catheter. When conduction passes directly under the tip of the catheter, the EGM will be very narrow and sharp, sometimes described as "near-field." Conduction seen at a distance from the catheter will result in an EGM that is wider and often not as sharp, which can be described as "far-field."

In this example, we are pacing in the CS. We have a Lasso catheter positioned inside a PV (*blue tracings*). Note that there are three distinct EGM morphologies in each of the four channels displayed.

Commentary: The *yellow arrow* points to the pacing spike. The *white arrow* points to near-field electrograms inside the PV and their characteristic near-field appearance. The *green arrow* points to far-field EGMs, which represent left atrial activity. Their morphology is considered far-field because they are recorded from within the PV. Since we are pacing in the CS, it is reasonable to expect that the Lasso catheter will "see" far-field left atrial activity before near-field PV activity.

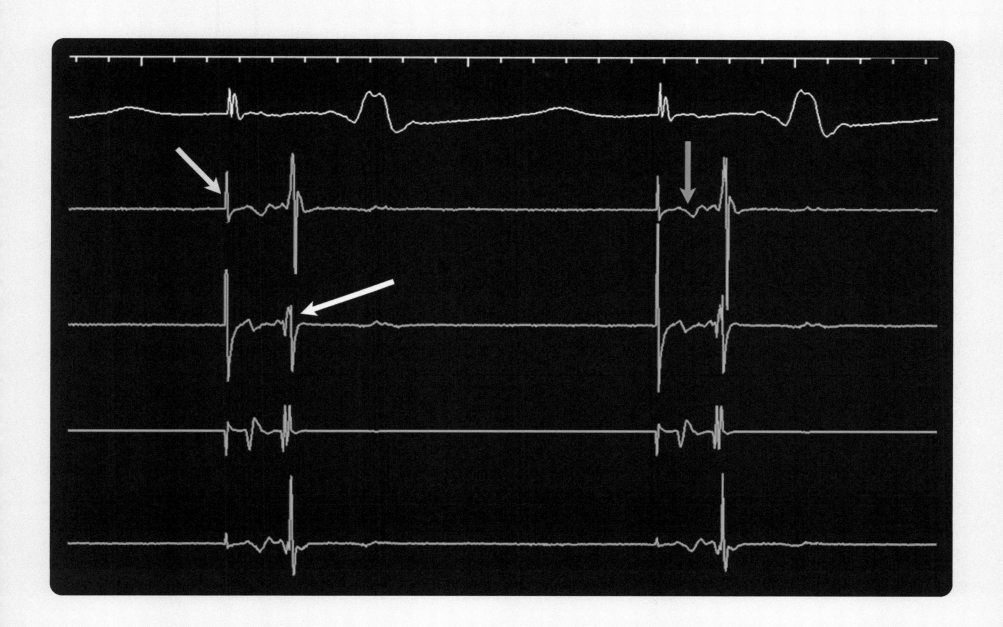

12. **Atrial Fibrillation** *continued*
Entrance Block

Entrance block refers to the absence of electrical conduction from the left atrium into the PVs. In this tracing, we are pacing the left atrium using CS 1-2. The *white arrows* indicate far-field EGMs recorded from the left atrium. The wave of depolarization successfully enters the PV (*first yellow arrow*) and gives rise to near-field PV potentials. A series of ablations are applied outside the PV in an attempt to separate it from the left atrium. During the last ablation lesion, as seen on the third beat, these local PV EGMs disappear (*third yellow arrow*). This indicates successful achievement of entrance block into that vein.

Also note the timing between the far-field left atrial potentials and the local PV potentials. The PV potentials got progressively later (see the first two beats) just before block occurred. The gradual progressive delay of these signals indicates the slowing of conduction into the PV as the ablation lesions are created. This is a great example of watching the EGMs "walk out" just before block occurs.

Commentary: The PV potentials will often demonstrate intermediate changes before conduction block is achieved. They tend to become progressively delayed with ongoing ablation. As well, activation sequence changes recorded on the Lasso catheter act as a guide to where in the PV antrum the next ablation lesion should be applied.

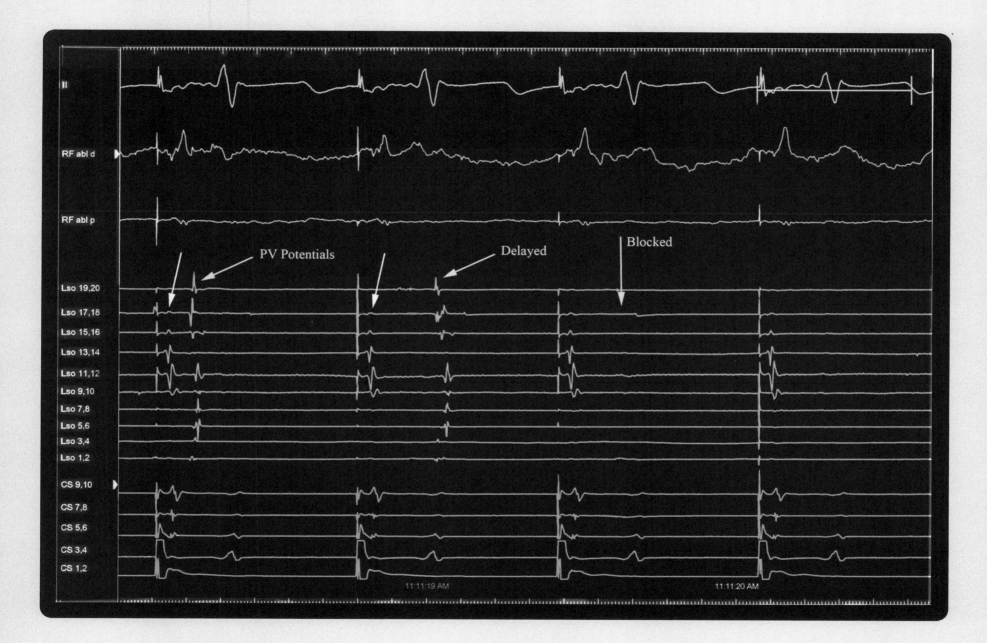

12. **Atrial Fibrillation** *continued*
Exit Block

In the case of PV ablation, exit block refers to conduction block in the opposite direction (ie, the absence of electrical conduction from within the PV to the left atrium). Theoretically, you may achieve exit block only or entrance block only (called unidirectional block). However, bidirectional block is our goal.

In this tracing, we are pacing the Lasso catheter positioned within a PV. The pacing spike has successfully captured the PV (see the small EGMs at the *arrows*). This demonstrates local capture within the PV.

Notice the surface ECG. It continues to show sinus rhythm uninterrupted by the pacing and capture within the PV. Also notice that the A and V signals on the CS catheter correspond to the surface P-wave and QRS, respectively. Therefore, we must have exit block. The local capture within the PV does not exit the PV and thus does not generate a P-wave on the surface ECG. If the PV had not been isolated, the local capture would have exited the PV into the left atrium and thus would have generated a P-wave on the surface ECG.

Combined with the previous tracing, we have confirmed bidirectional block in that vein.

Commentary: When pacing Lasso poles, it is often challenging to see local capture in the PV. Changing pacing poles will often solve this problem. When pacing the right PVs to test for exit block, pacing at high output may actually capture the right atrium and give the illusion of continued conduction even if exit block exists.

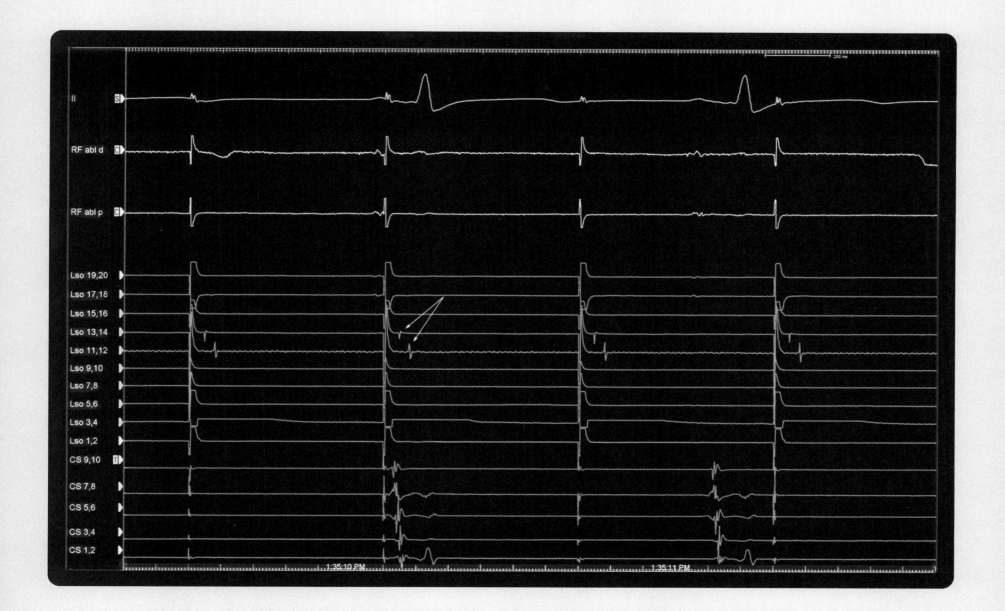

12. **Atrial Fibrillation** *continued*
Pulmonary Vein Fibrillation

This example reinforces the concept that successful ablation can "fence in" the electrical activity of the PVs and surrounding tissue, preventing exit into the atrium and initiation of AF. The blue Lasso signals here indicate that fibrillation is ongoing inside the PV. However, sinus rhythm continues (as seen on the surface ECG), unperturbed by the ongoing arrhythmia inside the vein.

In paroxysmal AF, the usual goal of ablation is electrical isolation of all four PVs to prevent ectopy in the veins from starting AF. In chronic AF, however, the ablation target is usually more complicated since the problem is not only the initiating beats from the veins but also the areas in the atrium that allow AF to persist.

In chronic AF, the first target is often isolation of the PVs. The second step is then some combination of ablating complex fractionated EGMs (CFEs), which are areas thought to contribute to sustaining the AF, as well as creating lines of conduction block in the left atrium across the roof and/or from mitral annulus to left PV (through the mitral isthmus). Another effect of creating these linear ablation lesion sets is to prevent flutter circuits from developing and the occurrence of left atrial flutter after the ablation. If a patient returns for a second ablation due to recurrent AF or left atrial flutter, the second procedure usually entails checking the veins for return of conduction, with further ablation applied to re-isolate them if necessary. If left atrial flutter is seen, then ablation is also directed at interrupting these circuits.

Commentary: Extra lines and targeting complex fractionated EGMs are all part of substrate modification. However, incomplete lines may, paradoxically, increase the substrate for left atrial flutter. Incomplete lines are worse than no lines at all. It is often very difficult to ablate patients returning with left atrial flutter because of the challenge in identifying the circuit and its critical zone.

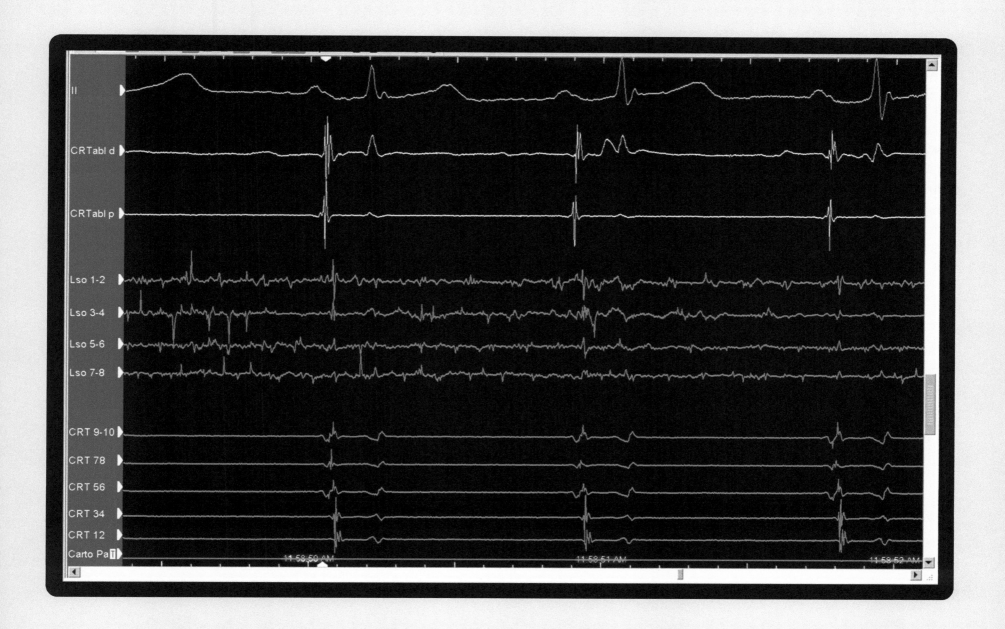

12. **Atrial Fibrillation** *continued*
Independent Pulmonary Vein Activity

Another sign of exit block from the PVs is sometimes seen without the need for pacing the Lasso catheter within the PV. Occasionally, following PV isolation, the PV may continue to have ectopy within it. This is a good example of PV independent activity.

For orientation, in this figure we have sinus rhythm on the surface ECG. The *yellow arrow* points to a far-field left atrial AEGM, and the *green arrow* points to a far-field VEGM. The *white arrows* point to independent activity within the PV that spontaneously generated a wave of depolarization within the PV but does not exit into the left atrium since no PACs are seen on the surface ECG.

Commentary: The foci within the PVs will not lead to AF due to exit block.

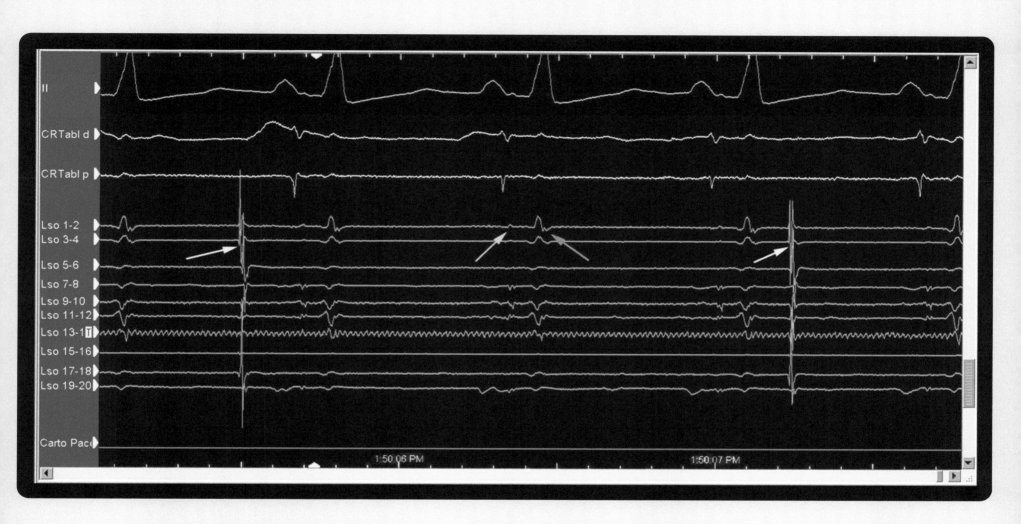

13. Ventricular Tachycardia
Basic Diagnosis

The SVTs discussed in the preceding pages are largely benign rhythms, although they can be highly symptomatic. In contrast, VT is an arrhythmia that originates in the ventricles and can be life-threatening. VT is most often associated with structural heart disease, such as prior myocardial infarction or poor ventricular function. Less commonly, VT can occur in structurally normal hearts.

On a 12-lead ECG, VT is recognized by its appearance as a wide-complex tachycardia. When a patient is having episodes of VT, acute management includes the basic principles of patient stabilization, such as assessing the "ABCs"—airway, breathing, and circulation. Treatment includes addressing reversible causes of VT, such as coronary heart disease or electrolyte disturbances, initiating anti-arrhythmic medications, and possibly inserting an implantable cardioverter–defibrillator. For selected patients with recurrent VT refractory to antiarrhythmic medications, an EP study and ablation can assist in decreasing the burden of VT.

Several strategies are used to localize and ablate VT:

- Activation mapping
- Pace mapping
- Entrainment mapping
- Substrate modification

Commentary: VT is a wide-complex tachycardia as seen on this 12-lead ECG. However, there are also other rhythms that can cause a wide-complex morphology, such as SVT with a bundle branch block, SVT using an AP, or paced rhythms. Careful examination of the QRS morphology and for the presence of P-waves on the ECG can often help distinguish between these diagnoses. In this example, the morphology of the QRS is most compatible with VT.

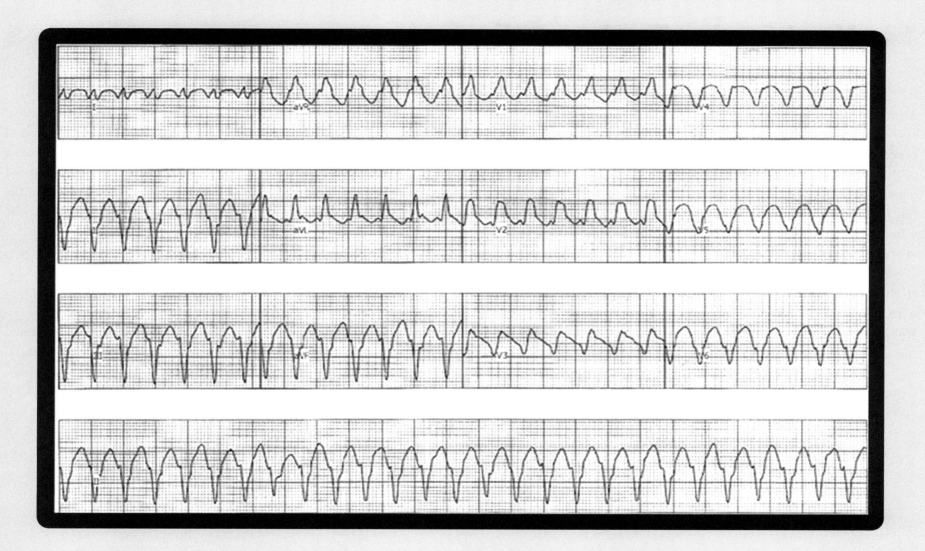

13. **Ventricular Tachycardia** *continued*
Activation Mapping

As previously described for activation mapping of atrial tachycardia, activation mapping is a strategy that can also be utilized for certain types of VT. This strategy involves recording of the relative timing of the ventricular depolarization in different areas of the ventricle, usually with the assistance of a 3D electroanatomic mapping system. Such a strategy is helpful when the VT is thought to originate from a focal point in the ventricle. In this situation, finding the earliest ventricular activity will identify the site of origin of the VT.

In this image, a shell representing the right ventricle was created with our 3D electroanatomic mapping system (Carto™, Biosense Webster) during VT. The color scheme is a visual representation of the activation sequence in the ventricle. Magenta represents areas with relatively late activation. Red represents areas with the earliest activation. The rainbow of colors represents intermediate areas of activation. In this example, the earliest activation is coming from a point source near the apex of the right ventricle. Therefore, the VT appears to be originating from the right ventricular apex where the activation is the earliest.

Commentary: Activation mapping is useful primarily when the mechanism of the VT is thought to be focal (when the VT is originating from a point source). In this situation, the earliest activation is the source of the VT. However, VT is often not focal but rather is caused by a reentrant circuit in the ventricle (more on this later). In this situation, activation mapping is not as helpful because the VT is caused by a loop or circuit of activation with no true beginning and no true end.

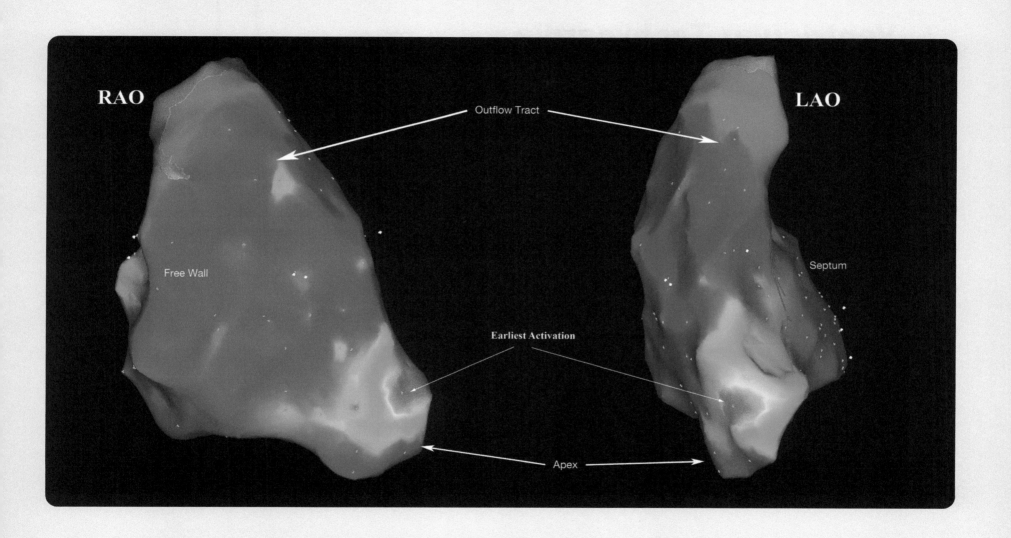

13. **Ventricular Tachycardia** *continued*
Pace Mapping

Pace mapping is a method that uses the QRS morphology on the ECG as a guide to locate the site of origin of the VT. This strategy is carried out using the catheter to pace several locations within the ventricle. The VT QRS morphology is studied, and there is an attempt to mimic the morphology of the clinical VT with that of the pacing morphology. This strategy is based on the concept that the QRS morphology of the VT will be reproduced by pacing the ventricle at the site of origin of the VT.

The ablation catheter is moved to different parts of the ventricle and pacing is performed. The closer the paced morphology matches the VT morphology, the closer the pacing site is to the origin or exit site of the VT. In this example, different locations in the right ventricular outflow tract were paced. The VT morphology is shown in the middle, and two different pacing sites are highlighted. One demonstrates a good morphology match, while the other shows a poor morphology match.

Commentary: Like all strategies, pace mapping has its pitfalls. One important factor is lead placement. Remember that in the EP lab, the ECG electrodes are often placed in nonconventional positions because the R2 (defibrillating) pads and ground patches prevent conventional lead placement. This can lead to dramatic changes in the apparent ECG morphology.

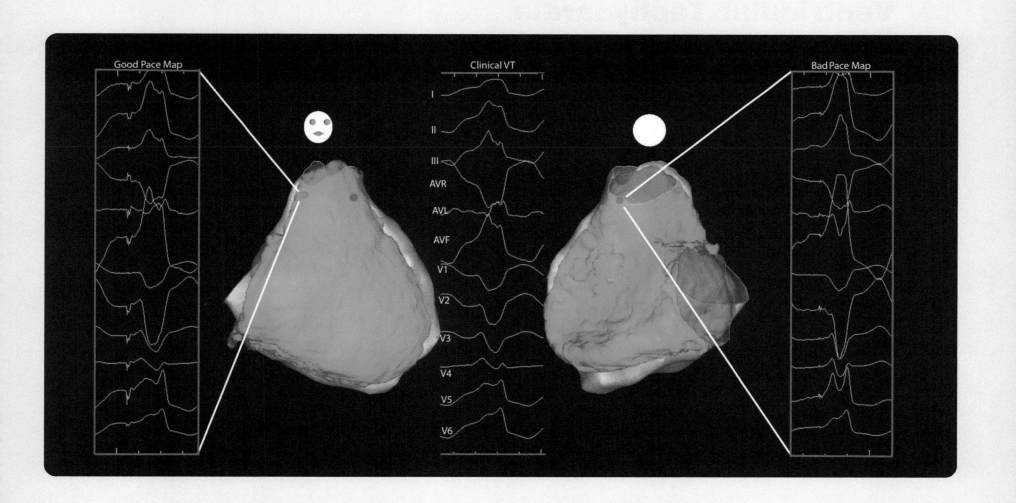

13. **Ventricular Tachycardia** *continued*
Entrainment Mapping

While activation mapping and pace mapping strategies are ideal for focal VTs, such strategies are less useful for VT caused by a large reentrant circuit. In this situation, entrainment maneuvers can be used to guide ablation. Entrainment is a difficult concept, and a comprehensive discussion is beyond the scope of this book.

However, the practical application of entrainment involves pacing the ventricle during VT at a slightly faster rate (eg, 20 to 30 msec) than the VT. If the VT persists following the paced beats, the response of the VT to the maneuver can give valuable information. The VT morphology during the pacing maneuver and the length of the interval following the last paced beat (the PPI) are two of the characteristics that are studied. This information can help ascertain whether the pacing site is within a critical portion of the VT circuit that may be a good target for ablation.

Commentary: Here are examples of entrainment of the same VT from two different pacing sites. Note that in both examples, the VT is accelerated slightly with pacing and that the VT persists following the pacing maneuver. The PPI has been measured in the ablation channel since it was the catheter we used for pacing. The PPI is the time from the last paced beat to the first EGM of the persisting VT.

Without going through the complexities of entrainment, the top panel shows a PPI that is long compared with the cycle length of the VT. The bottom panel shows a PPI that is essentially the same as the cycle length of the VT. When the PPI is relatively long, the pacing site is not a part of the VT circuit. When the PPI is similar to that of the VT cycle length, the pacing site is a within the VT circuit and may be an area of interest to ablate.

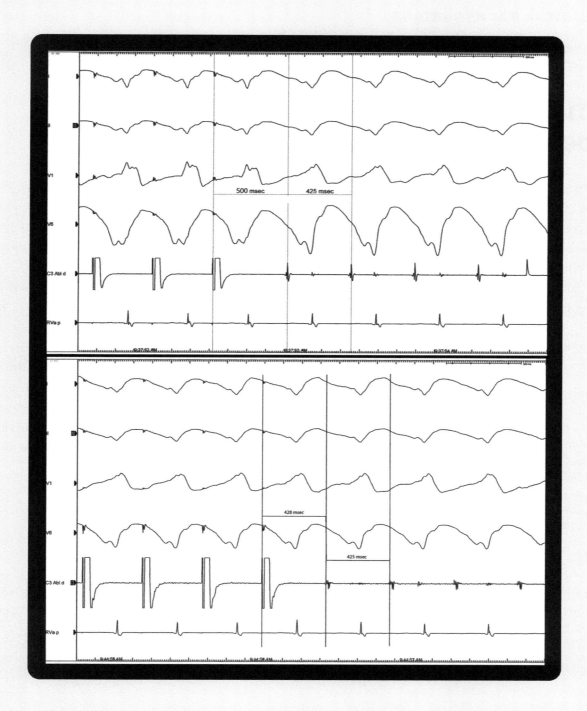

13. Ventricular Tachycardia *continued*
Scar-dependent Ventricular Tachycardia

VT associated with structural heart disease is often dependent on the presence of scar tissue. Areas of scar tissue contain myocardial cells that have various degrees of damage. Some cells are completely dead and are a part of true scar that is unable to depolarize. Other cells are damaged but are still alive and able to depolarize, although conduction through these cells can be very slow. Typically, damaged areas of myocardium are zones of slow conduction that can give rise to reentrant VT circuits.

This image presents a simplified representation of scar within the ventricular myocardium. Note the paths of slowly conducting cells within the scar tissue. These areas of slowly conducting cells can form a circuit (as depicted by the *arrows*), which gives rise to a reentrant VT.

With successful targeted ablation of slowly conducting cells within or adjacent to the scar, VT circuits are less likely to form.

Commentary: Any peri-infarct zone has the ability to slowly conduct a wave of depolarization into the surrounding healthy myocardium. This image illustrates one exit site. However, there may be many exit sites along the peri-infarct zone. Ablating one site may only reveal a secondary exit site that will change the VT morphology.

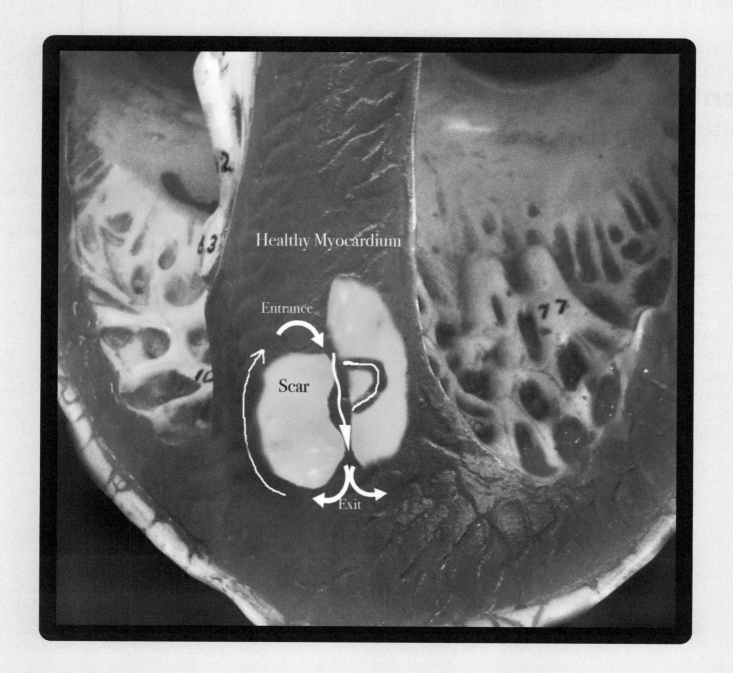

13. **Ventricular Tachycardia** *continued*
Voltage Mapping

The purpose of voltage mapping is to identify healthy versus scarred heart tissue and the transition zone between these two areas. In patients with structural heart disease, myocardial damage (following a myocardial infarction, for example) creates areas of scar that can be the substrate for VT caused by a reentrant circuit. By identifying the scar, the locations of possible VT circuits are ascertained.

Voltage mapping is performed using a 3D electroanatomic mapping system. The mapping catheter is moved to different locations in the ventricles, and the amplitude of the associated EGM is noted. The computerized mapping system generates a visual representation of the ventricle and depicts large, healthy EGMs as magenta. Small EGMs likely representing scar are shown in red. Transition zones are depicted by a rainbow pattern.

Commentary: The color scheme is simply a visual representation of the collected EGM information. By convention, EGMs larger than 1.5 mV (*yellow arrow*) are usually set as magenta, EGMs smaller than 0.5 mV are set as red (*green arrow*), and EGMs between 0.5 and 1.5 mV are set as a rainbow gradient.

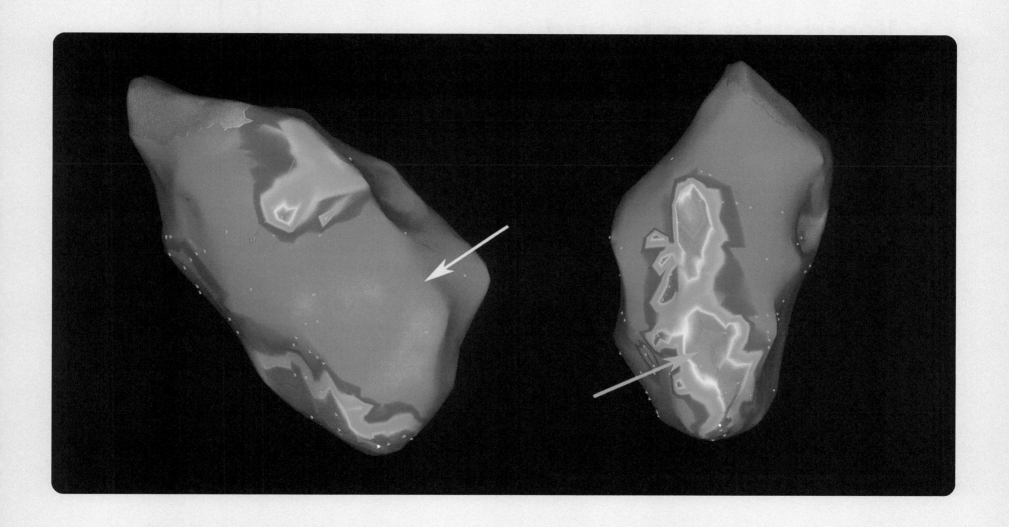

13. Ventricular Tachycardia *continued*
Substrate Modification

Substrate modification is an anatomic-based, empiric ablation approach that does not focus on mapping the location of a specific VT. Instead, the strategy is based on finding the areas in the ventricle that are most susceptible to maintaining a VT circuit and attempting to ablate such areas. The principle is that VT circuits form in areas of damaged but living heart tissue. An attempt is made to ablate the damaged tissue so that it can no longer be involved in forming VT circuits.

Substrate modification is therefore an empiric ablation strategy that is used for VT when the VT is non-inducible or not hemodynamically tolerated. In this setting, it is not possible to use other strategies such as pace mapping, activation mapping, or entrainment mapping. Areas of scar are identified by creating a voltage map, as described previously. The hallmark of scar includes low-voltage and/or fractionated EGMs. Often, the damaged tissue responsible for the VT circuit involves the border zones of the scar.

Commentary: This figure shows two views of a 3D electroanatomic map of the left ventricle. The color scheme has been set to visually represent the size of the VEGMs at various sites. The red areas represent scar, whereas the magenta areas represent healthy tissue. The intermediary rainbow colors represent the border zone of scar. In this case, the scar was modified by placing ablation lesions (*red dots*) around the border zone.

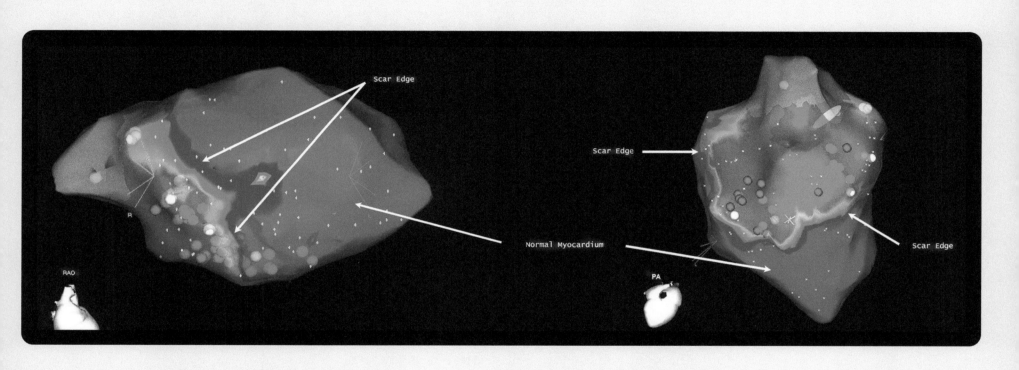

Unit 3:
Advanced Concepts

This unit examines some slightly more advanced concepts, including the use of unipolar leads, additional EP principles such as gap phenomenon and latency, and diagnostic maneuvers such as delivering premature ventricular contractions (PVCs) into tachycardia, tachycardia entrainment, and para-Hisian pacing.

Understanding these concepts will increase your understanding of cardiac EP and the mechanisms of tachycardias.

Commentary: The tracing here, hidden within the nebula, is a PVC that has been delivered during AVNRT. See page 106 for more details.

UNIT 3 OUTLINE

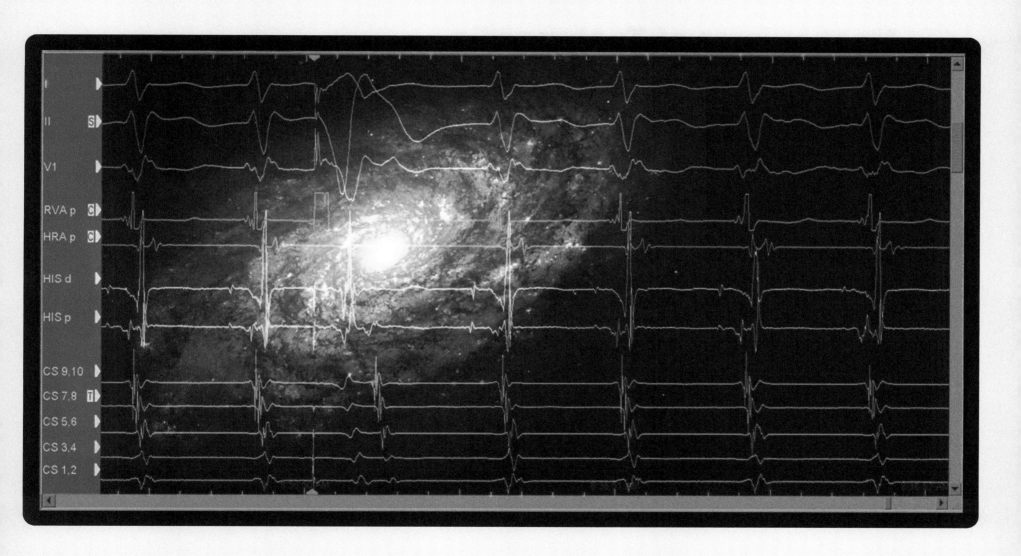

14. Mechanisms of Tachycardia

Tachycardias are caused by one of three underlying mechanisms: reentry, enhanced automaticity, and triggered activity. Conceptually, it helps to categorise these mechanisms into one of two major categories:

- Macro-reentrant circuits
- Focal tachycardias

Macro reentry is essentially a self-perpetuating loop of electrical activity that often incorporates a large area of the atrium, ventricle, or both. In a reentrant circuit, there is a leading "head" of depolarization and a trailing "tail" of recovery where the head is constantly chasing the tail (depicted by the *circular black arrows*). Examples include atrial flutter, AVNRT, and AVRT. These tachycardias require a zone of fast conduction and a zone of slow conduction.

In contrast, focal tachycardias emanate from a point source in the heart (depicted by the *green star*) and are not dependent on a large circuit of electrical activity. A typical example of a focal tachycardia is atrial tachycardia. Two possible mechanisms of a focal tachycardia are automaticity and triggered activity, both of which lead to abnormal spontaneous depolarizations of a myocardial cell.

Automaticity is a normal property of some specialized cells such as the sinus node. Automaticity can be an unexpected property in abnormal cells such as those found in a focal atrial tachycardia. Triggered activity is the abnormal spontaneous depolarization of cells during or immediately following the normal recovery period of the cell (called "after-depolarizations"). Triggered activity can be initiated by excess calcium in the cell.

Commentary: The mechanism of the tachycardia is relevant to the EP study because it affects the manner in which the tachycardia is induced and studied. Macro-reentrant rhythms are more readily induced using extra-stimuli pacing, whereas triggered or automatic rhythms are less readily induced using pacing maneuvers.

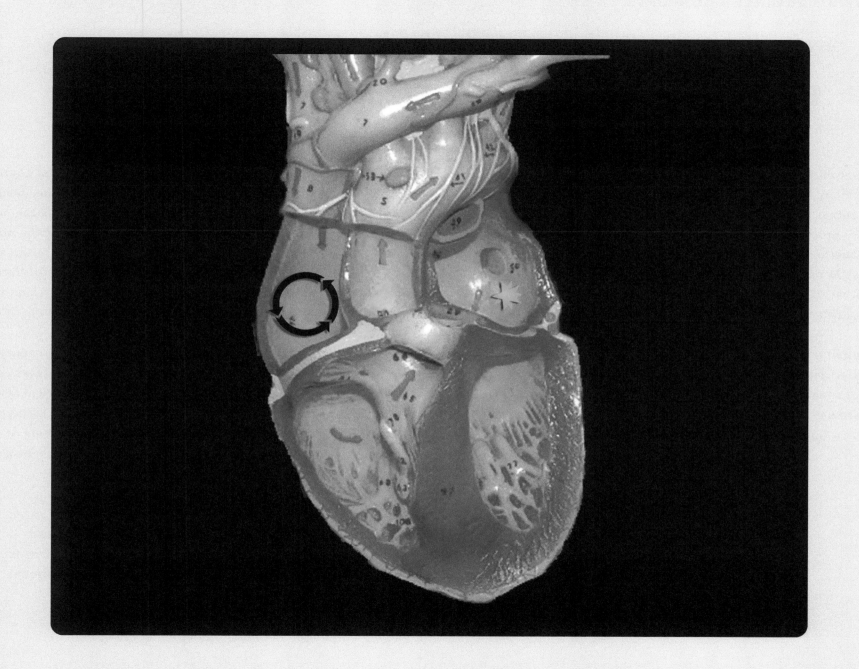

15. Bipolar Versus Unipolar Electrograms

By convention, most of the intracardiac EGMs are bipolar recordings. However, there are differences between unipolar and bipolar recordings that can be exploited. A bipolar recording refers to the use of two poles (a positive and negative electrode) in close proximity to one another. A unipolar recording must also use two poles to generate an EGM but refers to the use of a single pole (by convention, the positive electrode) in contact with the area of interest and a distant second electrode (by convention, the negative electrode).

A unipolar EGM tends to represent more of a global picture of the cardiac depolarization, whereas a bipolar EGM tends to represent depolarization in a specific area (between the two bipoles). Since we are usually primarily interested in the timing of local electrical activity, bipolar EGMs are generally recorded.

However, specific situations, such as mapping for a point source of activity, can call for unipolar recordings. For example, when mapping for a left-sided AP, the mapping catheter is moved along the mitral annulus. As the ventricle is paced, the earliest part of the atrium to be activated localizes the AP. This figure shows the mitral valve as seen from the left atrium. The unipolar EGM is useful because any electrical activity propagating in a direction toward a unipolar recording pole will create a positive deflection (an R-wave).

Any electrical activity propagating away from a unipolar recording pole will create a negative deflection (a Q-wave). Only when the catheter tip is placed at the site of the AP will all electrical activity emanate away from the unipolar electrode (*green arrows*). Therefore, when the unipolar EGM begins with a Q-wave, this suggests that the catheter is at the source of earliest activity and will likely be a good target to ablate.

Commentary: A unipolar lead is just a very wide bipolar lead. The positive electrode is the tip of the catheter. The negative pole is usually Wilson's central terminal. It can also be an indifferent electrode in the inferior vena cava.

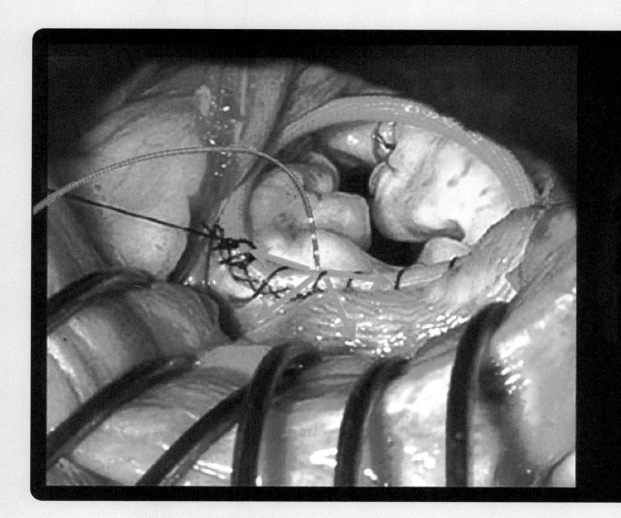

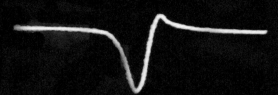

Unipolar EGM initiating with a Q-wave

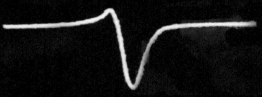

Unipolar EGM initiating with an R-wave

16. Latency

With respect to pacing, the latent period is defined as the time period between delivery of the pacing stimulus and the local depolarization of the myocardium. Typically, the latent period is very small and the local depolarization immediately follows the pacing stimulus. An increase in latency refers to an increase in the delay of local capture of the myocardium from a paced impulse.

Latency increases when the pacing cycle length approaches the absolute refractory period of the myocardial cells. For example, when an S2 is delivered very tightly coupled to the last S1, there is an increased delay before the resulting EGM is seen. In this figure, the *orange arrow* indicates local capture immediately after the pacing spike during the S1 drive train. The *green arrow* points to the local capture following the S2. Notice that the time delay between the pacing spike and the EGM is much longer.

Commentary: There are two relevant consequences of latency. The first is that when increasing latency is seen, one can expect that with slightly shorter coupling intervals the myocardium will likely lose capture. In other words, the coupling interval is approaching the absolute refractory period of the myocardial cells.

The second consequence is that the latency period affects the EP response of the heart. For example, when delivering an atrial extra-stimulus with a coupling interval of 600-300 msec, due to increased latency after the S2, the atrium may only capture at a coupling interval of 600-310 msec (ie, 10 msec of latency). This delay in atrial depolarization, although apparently minor, can lead to effects such as the gap phenomenon described on the next page.

Furthermore, the delay also affects the measurement of intervals. For example, when attempting to measure the ERP of the AV node, the pacing stimulus may be delivered at 600-300 msec, but this interval is not relevant to the AV node. What is relevant to the AV node is the coupling interval of the atrial depolarization reaching the AV node. Differences between the S1 and S2 with respect to latency and other factors, such as delay in transatrial conduction time, may result in atrial depolarization at the AV node of 600-315 msec. Therefore, if the AV node blocks with this delivered extra-stimulus, the ERP of the node is not 600-300 msec. Rather, it is 600-315 msec.

Always measure the ERP of any structure using the catheter closest to that structure!

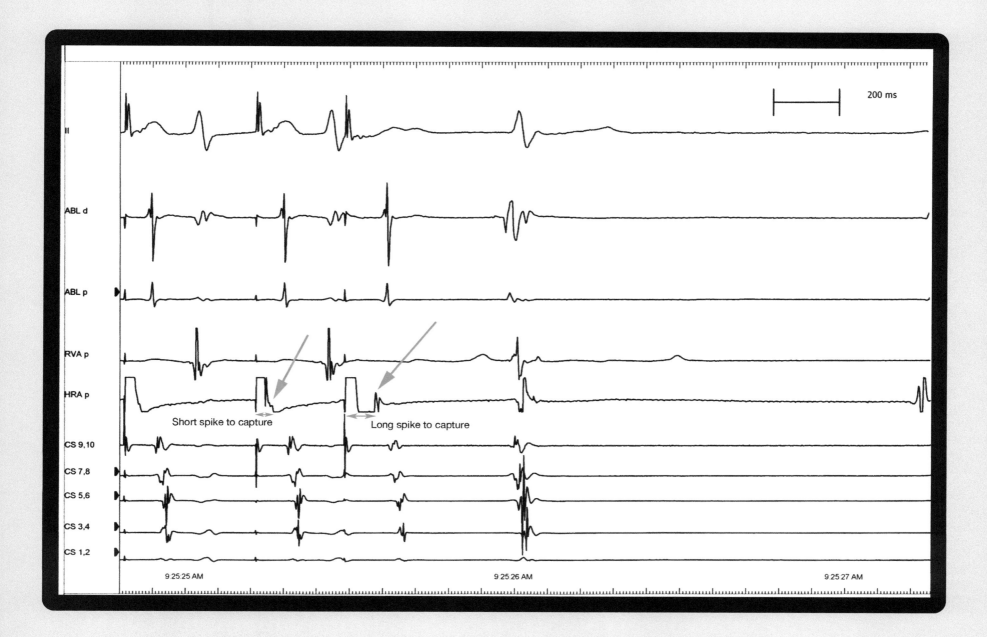

II

ABL d

ABL p

RVA p

HRA p

Short spike to capture   Long spike to capture

CS 9,10

CS 7,8

CS 5,6

CS 3,4

CS 1,2

200 ms

9:25:25 AM   9:25:26 AM   9:25:27 AM

17. Gap Phenomenon

Gap phenomenon refers to the observation of unexpected resumption of conduction when delivering incrementally shorter S1-S2 coupled extra-stimuli. It is a phenomenon that can be seen in any tissue but was first observed during the testing of AV nodal conduction using a single extra-stimulus. This figure demonstrates an example of gap phenomenon. In the left panel, the AV node does not conduct to the ventricle with a coupling interval of 600-300 msec—the ERP of the AV node has been reached. However, as shorter coupling intervals were incrementally delivered, unexpected resumption of AV nodal conduction occurred at 600-270 msec (right panel). How does this occur?

Gap phenomenon occurs because the coupling of the pacing stimuli (S1-S2) does not necessarily reflect the received coupling interval of the conducting myocardial tissue (AV node). The presence of conduction delay related to the S2 can paradoxically increase the received coupling interval at the level of previous block and thus conduction may resume.

This complicated phenomenon is best described by example. When pacing from the right atrium and testing AV nodal conduction, as shown here, delay can manifest from two main sources: latency and intra-atrial conduction delay.

As mentioned earlier, latency refers to local delay in myocardial capture (*arrow*). This local delay translates into a lengthening of the effective coupling interval that is delivered to the AV node.

Intra-atrial conduction time refers to the time for conduction to transit from the atrial pacing site to the AV node. While generally fixed, intra-atrial conduction time can lengthen at tight coupling intervals, also causing lengthening of the effective coupling interval delivered to the AV node. When the delay is long enough to allow the refractory period of the AV node to pass, AV nodal conduction may resume.

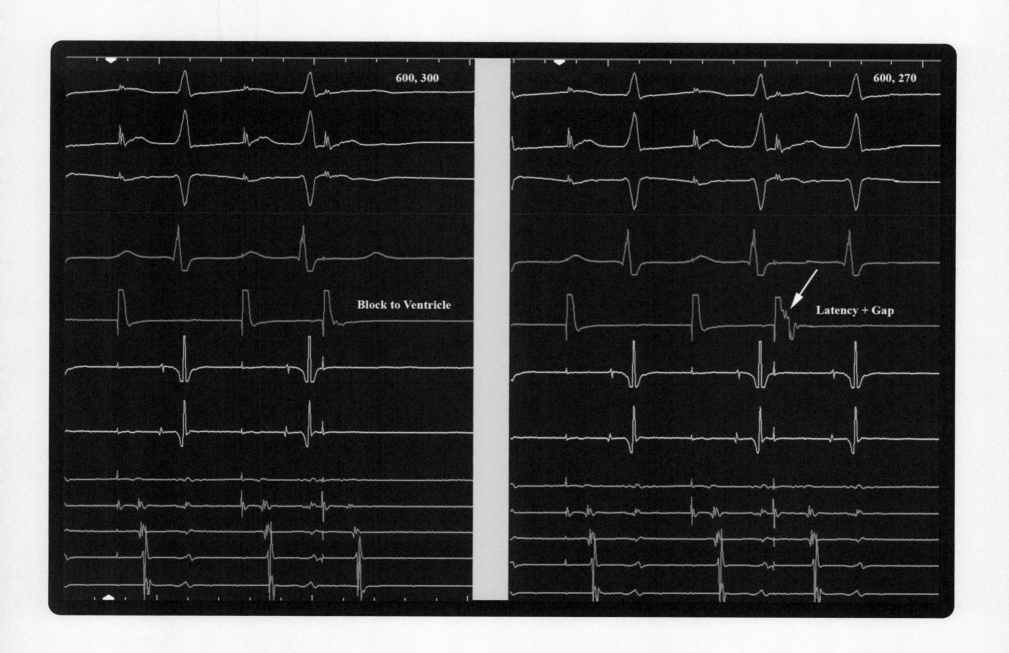

18. PVCs into AVNRT

When an SVT is induced during an EP study, various diagnostic maneuvers can be performed to assist in diagnosing the SVT. One helpful maneuver is the introduction of ventricular extra-stimuli (PVCs or S2s) into the tachycardia beginning slightly faster than the TCL. The response of a ventricular extra-stimulus during AVNRT is explained here; see the next page for an explanation of the response during AVRT.

As previously described, AVNRT is a small reentrant circuit in the AV node. By delivering PVCs from the ventricle, it is generally difficult to penetrate such a small circuit and conduct to the atrium. Therefore, the atrial cycle length is not often affected by the ventricular extra-stimulus.

In this figure, the diagnosis of AVRT is already excluded because the V-A time is too short; therefore, AVNRT is the likely diagnosis. With delivery of the ventricular extra-stimulus, the subsequent AEGM is not affected and remains at the TCL (380 msec).

Commentary: In this example, the diagnosis of AVNRT was already known prior to the pacing maneuver. However, the ventricular extra-stimulus during AVNRT has a second purpose. During AVNRT, the AEGM and VEGM are often superimposed. Therefore, it is difficult to analyze the atrial activation sequence. By stimulating the ventricle early, the VEGM no longer overlaps the AEGM and the true atrial activation sequence can be analyzed properly. Determining whether the atrial activation is earliest on the HIS catheter (anterior, *arrow*) versus the proximal CS catheter (posterior) is helpful for the physician in judging the risk of inadvertently ablating the AV nodal fast pathway.

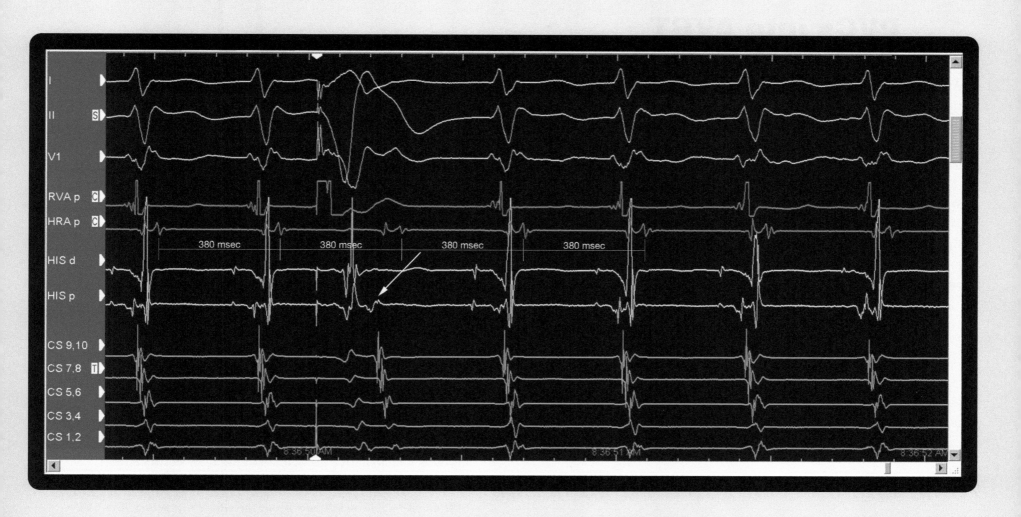

19. PVCs into AVRT

As opposed to AVNRT (see previous page), the introduction of a PVC into AVRT commonly affects the atrium. Because the reentrant circuit of AVRT is relatively large, a PVC has relatively easy access to the tachycardia circuit, and this can affect the timing or presence of the subsequent AEGM.

When a PVC is delivered at the same time as or just before an expected HIS signal (called a "His-refractory PVC"), the response can be highly informative. This maneuver is used to assess the presence of an AP and determine whether the AP is an active participant in the tachycardia.

Commentary: When a His-refractory PVC is introduced into an SVT, there are several possible responses:

1. The tachycardia continues and the subsequent atrial cycle length is unaffected. This is the least informative response. This response would be expected with AVNRT since the atrium cannot be affected because the His (or AV node) is refractory. However, AVRT is not excluded by this response.

2. The tachycardia continues and the subsequent atrial cycle length becomes earlier (the atrium is "advanced"). This proves the *presence* of an AP. A PVC introduced while the His is refractory cannot affect the atrium unless there is a secondary route to the atrium (ie, an AP). However, this response does not confirm that the AP is necessarily participating in the tachycardia. This figure demonstrates what we call "advancing the next A."

3. The tachycardia continues and the subsequent atrial cycle length becomes later or "delayed." When the tachycardia slows down because of the PVC, this can only be explained by slowed conduction through the AP ("decremental" properties) and proves it is an active participant in the tachycardia circuit.

4. The tachycardia terminates *without* conduction to the atrium. When a PVC is introduced while the His is refractory, the PVC has no way to affect the AV node. If the PVC does not conduct to the atrium, it cannot affect an atrial tachycardia. Therefore, a His-refractory PVC that terminates the tachycardia without conducting the atrium proves AVRT (by exclusion).

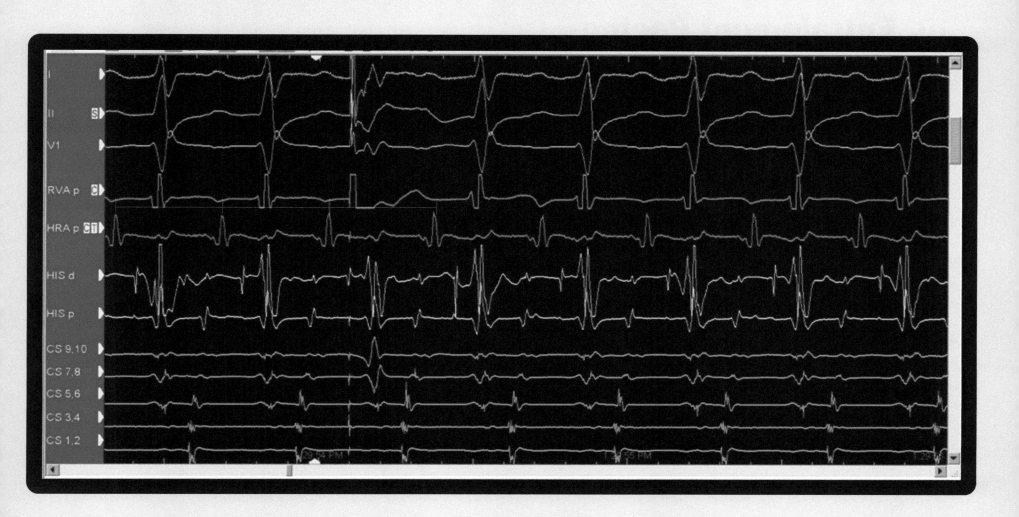

20. Entrainment Pacing

"Entrainment" of a tachycardia refers to a specific response of a macro-reentrant tachycardia to a pacing rate that is slightly faster than the tachycardia. This complex concept was superficially discussed on page 88. The main purpose of entrainment is to determine the proximity of the pacing catheter to the tachycardia circuit.

During tachycardia, an attempt can be made to entrain the tachycardia by pacing at a cycle length that is slightly shorter (10 to 20 msec) than the TCL. The goal is to penetrate the tachycardia circuit, speed it up to the pacing rate, and then stop pacing and observe the response. Once pacing is stopped, the timing of the first return EGM in the pacing channel typically provides important information.

The interval between the last pacing stimulus and the first return EGM (measured in the pacing channel) is the PPI. For this measurement to be useful, the pacing must not terminate the tachycardia. Simply, the longer the PPI, the farther away the pacing catheter is from the tachycardia circuit. The shorter the PPI (the closer the PPI approximates the TCL), the closer the pacing catheter is to the tachycardia circuit.

This figure shows an example of AVNRT, entrained from the right ventricular apical catheter. Keep in mind how far away the RVA catheter is from the AVNRT circuit. Once pacing is stopped, the PPI is measured (*white arrow*) and compared with the TCL (*yellow arrow*). The PPI is relatively long, suggesting that the RVA catheter is far from the tachycardia circuit. This finding is expected and compatible with AVNRT.

Commentary: In contrast, if the tachycardia had been an example of AVRT, the RVA catheter would be in much closer proximity to the tachycardia circuit (which involves the atrium, the AV node, the ventricle, and the AP). In this situation, the PPI would be shorter. Studies have shown that a PPI–TCL difference of 115 msec is a useful cutoff to differentiate AVNRT (>115 msec) and AVRT (<115 msec) due to the principles explained above. The principle of entrainment can be used for any macro-reentrant tachycardia. However, there are pitfalls to entrainment that are beyond the scope of this text. The example here illustrates its use in an SVT. Its use in VT mapping was demonstrated on page 88.

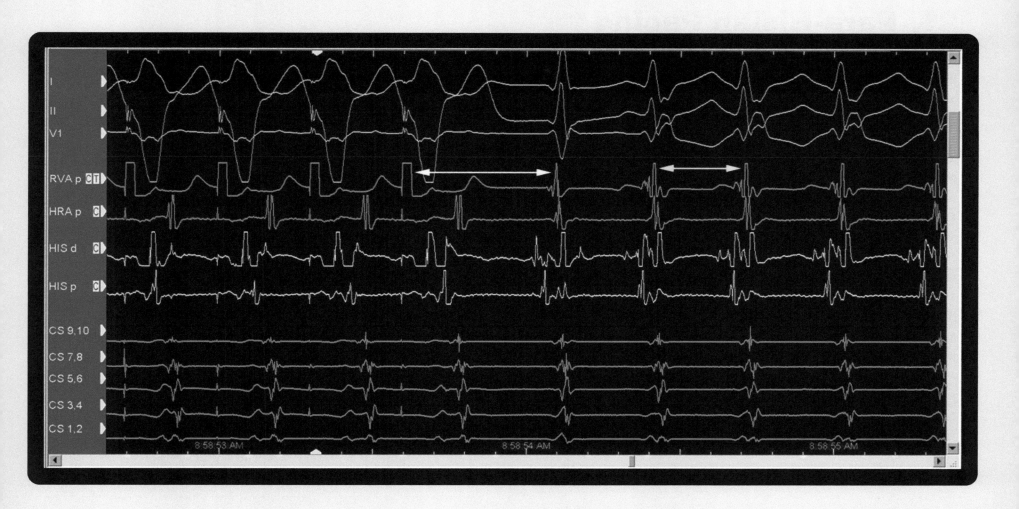

21. Para-Hisian Pacing

When an AP is located away from the septum, the diagnosis is usually obvious due to the abnormal atrial activation sequence during ventricular pacing. However, when the AP is located close to the septum (near the AV node), the diagnosis is less obvious because it is difficult to differentiate between retrograde AV nodal conduction and retrograde AP conduction.

The "para-Hisian" pacing maneuver was developed to assist in the diagnosis of septal APs. Para-Hisian pacing refers to pacing beside or close to the bundle of His (*para* = beside or next to). The performance of this maneuver involves two steps: pacing near the His bundle at a high output (which captures the HIS signal) and pacing near the His bundle at a low output (which only captures the para-Hisian myocardium).

- **Step 1** (high output): The catheter is placed near the His bundle (large His potential should be seen). Since the His bundle is protected by the surrounding myocardium, a higher output (typically 20 mA) is required to capture the His signal. His bundle capture is diagnosed when the QRS is narrow since the ventricles are depolarized normally through the specialized His-Purkinje system.

- **Step 2** (low output): The pacing output is then decreased until capture of the His bundle is lost but the output is still sufficient to capture the adjacent myocardium. Myocardial capture is diagnosed by a widening of the QRS since the ventricle is now being paced without the use of the specialized His-Purkinje system.

Capturing the His bundle during high-output pacing will generate a relatively short V-A time (measured from the pacing stimulus to the atrial signal) since the wave of depolarization will travel retrogradely through the AV node and into the atrium directly.

At low output and loss of His capture, the V-A interval will depend on whether a septal AP is present. When no septal AP is present, capturing the myocardium generates a much longer V-A time since the stimulus captures only local ventricular myocardium. The wave of depolarization needs to reach the Purkinje system near the apex of the ventricle then travel up the bundle branches and finally retrogradely through the AV node. The difference in V-A time between His bundle capture and ventricular-only capture should be approximately 45 to 50 msec.

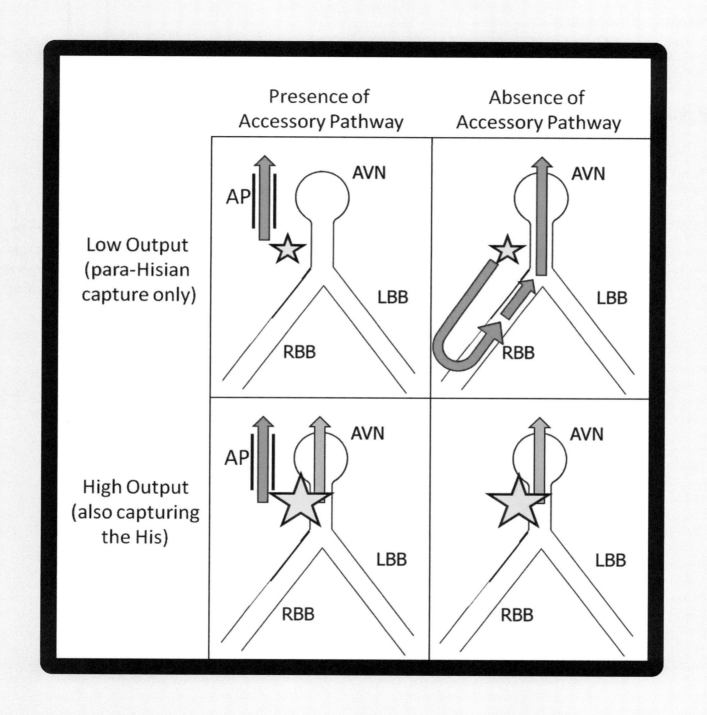

21. **Para-Hisian Pacing** *continued*

This is an example of an AV nodal response.

Commentary: Note the difference in length of the blue arrows. The difference in V-A time between ventricular capture (*first blue arrow*, with wide QRS [*white arrow*]) and His capture (*second blue arrow*, with narrow QRS [*yellow arrow*]) is approximately 70 msec.

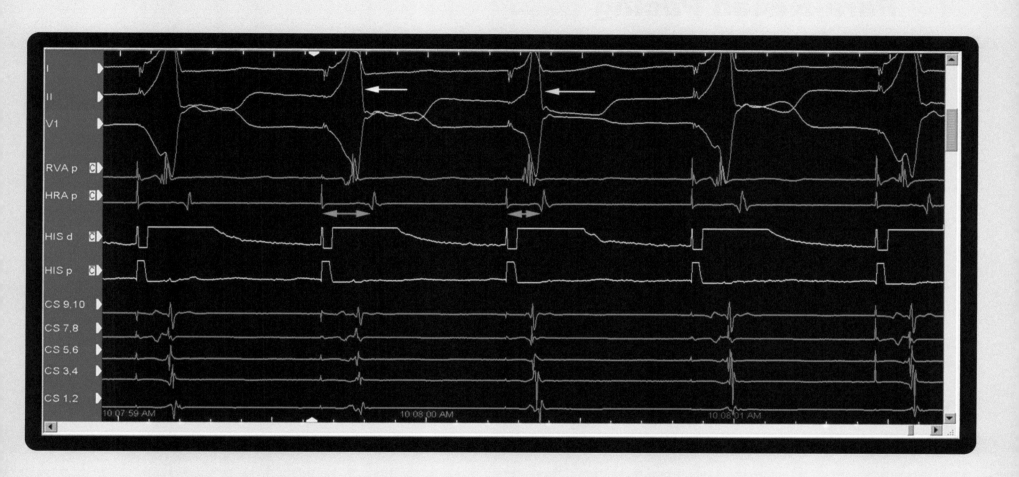

21. **Para-Hisian Pacing** *continued*

This is an example of an anteroseptal AP response.

Commentary: If a septal pathway is present, the V-A times are essentially identical since the AP yields a direct path to the atrium regardless of whether the His bundle is captured. In this example, the difference in V-A time between HIS capture (123 msec, with narrow QRS) and ventricular capture (119 msec, with wide QRS) is indicated.

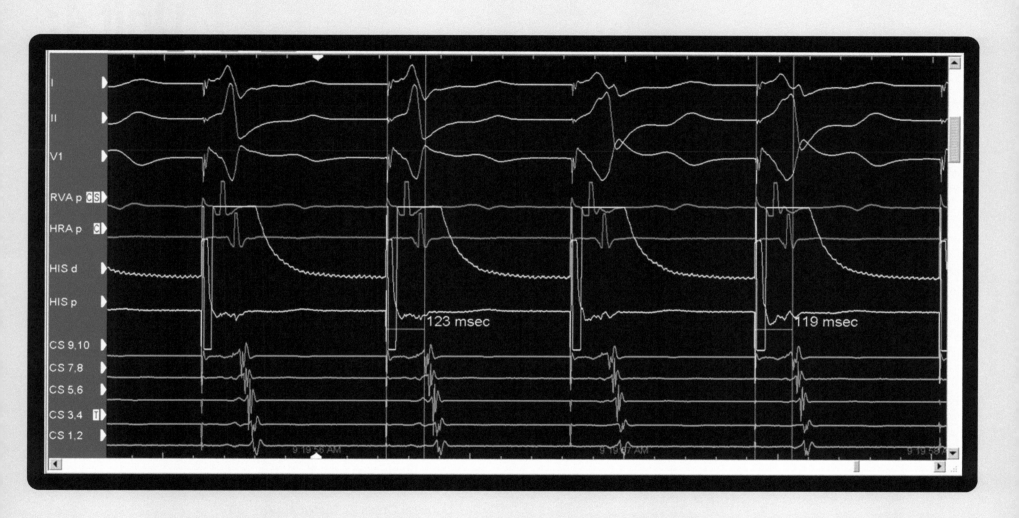

Unit 4:
Advanced Tracings

In this unit we present some representative tracings illustrating the thinking process that one uses during the course of the study. Correct interpretation requires both a fundamental knowledge of facts and the ability to use them in deductive reasoning. The learning process is life-long and this is but a small sampling.

There are other points of interest that are not discussed and even other possible explanations. Some issues are quite black and white, while others may be more open to alternate explanations or speculation. Try to sort out this tracing before reading the commentary. In this tracing, a premature atrial beat (*arrow*) is programmed into the tachycardia. What is the mechanism of this tachycardia?

Commentary: This is a "wide-complex" tachycardia, a common clinical interpretative dilemma. The differential diagnosis includes VT, SVT with bundle branch block aberrancy, and SVT with pre-excitation (WPW).

There is one atrial deflection for each ventricular deflection, but one does not know whether it is an SVT leading the QRS or a VT conducting retrogradely to the atrium. The HIS catheter, properly positioned, does not show a His bundle deflection, ruling out SVT with aberrancy. This leaves VT or pre-excited tachycardia.

If you caliper carefully, you will see that this PAC advances the next QRS. This would not be expected with VT, where a change in the ventricular timing after a PAC would be very rare. You might ponder why this is so. We are now only left with the correct diagnosis of pre-excited antidromic tachycardia.

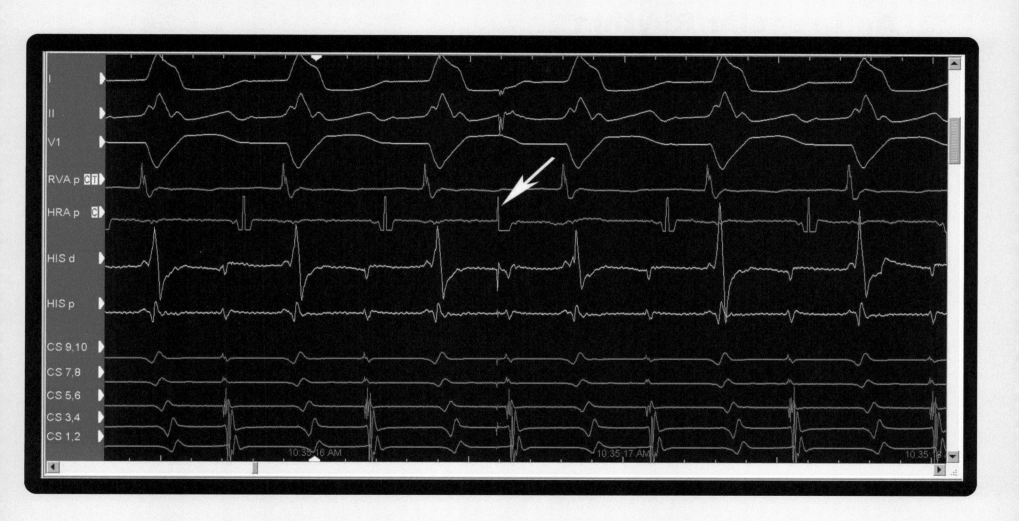

22. An Irregular Rhythm

The rhythm shown here is relatively slow and irregular. What is happening?

Commentary: The first, second, and last cycles have no preceding atrial activity. The QRS is narrow and atrial activation is essentially simultaneous with the QRS. This is most compatible with a junctional rhythm that probably originates within the AV node/His bundle region and is a common escape rhythm with sinus bradycardia. The third and fourth beats are preceded by atrial activity and a surface P-wave. Atrial activity begins in the distal CS (1-2). These are most compatible with PACs coming from the left atrium, possibly as a result of pressure from the CS catheter.

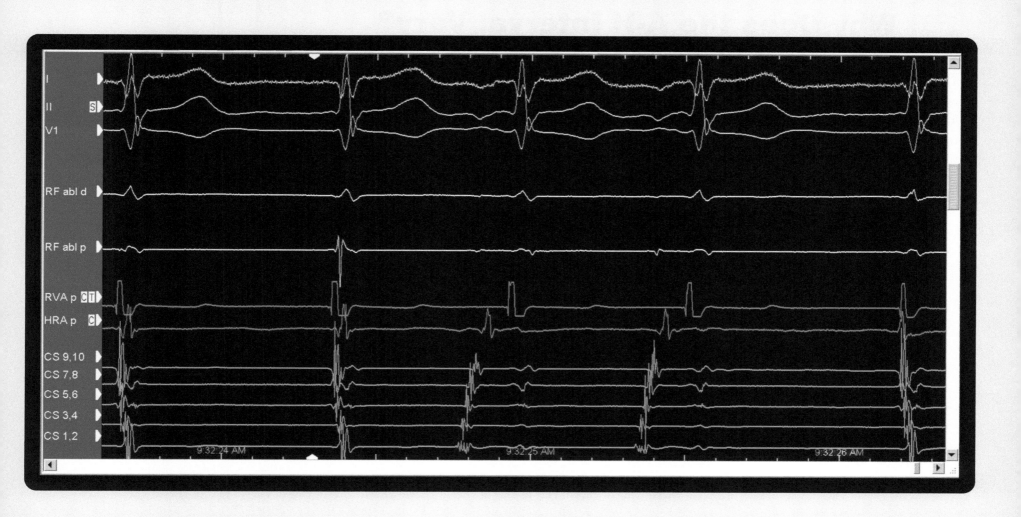

23. Why Does the A-H Interval Vary?

This figure shows the last two beats of a drive (S1). The A-H interval is prolonged after the premature stimulus S2 since it is early and AV nodal conduction is rate-dependent. However, it shortens again after the second extra-stimulus, the S3. One might expect it to prolong even further after a second extra-stimulus.

Commentary: The critical factor determining the subsequent A-H interval is the length of the preceding cycle. In this example, even though the S3 is the second in a row, it is coming after a relatively long interval between the S2 and S3, allowing the AV node to recover from refractoriness. The A-H interval will surely shorten as the interval between S2 and S3 lengthens.

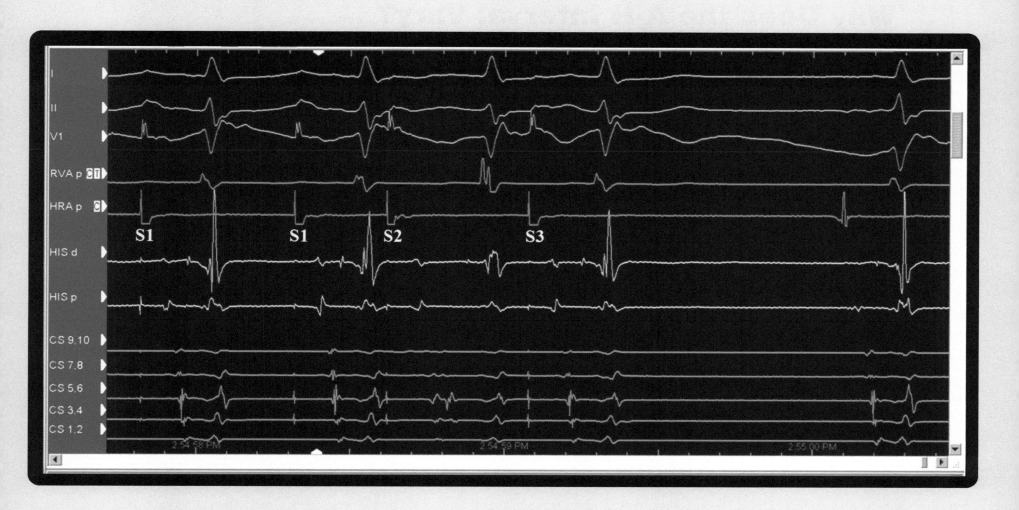

23. **Why Does the A-H Interval Vary?** *continued*

In this tracing, we tried inducing an SVT with a ventricular extra-stimulus (S2). It blocked in the left lateral AP as well as the AV node. However, a spontaneous PVC did successfully initiate AVRT. Each QRS during tachycardia is followed closely by eccentric atrial activation starting in the distal CS (1-2). This can only be AVRT over a left lateral AP (you may consider why). Interestingly, the TCL is irregular, which is related to a changing A-H interval. Why is the A-H interval changing?

Commentary: The concept of dual AV nodal pathways has been discussed, and the slow AV nodal pathway is usually the antegrade limb of the circuit in AVNRT. However, patients with A-V tachycardias may also have dual pathways.

In this example, antegrade conduction utilizes either the slow pathway or the fast pathway with some decrement. Since the right ventricular PVC takes much longer to travel to the AP, the A-H interval is shorter. Once the tachycardia is under way, the circuit is smaller, shortening the A-A time and thus lengthening the A-H interval.

In such patients, dual AV nodal pathways may also manifest AVNRT as well as AVRT.

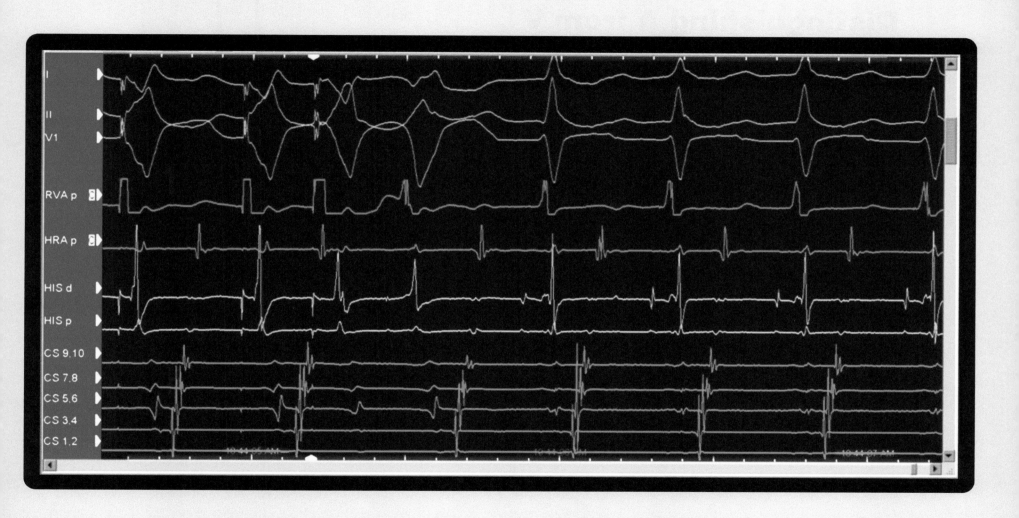

24. Distinguishing A from V

In this tracing, one sees the last paced beat of an atrial drive (S1) and the atrial extra-stimulus (S2). The A-H interval after the S2 is longer than after the S1 and is sufficiently long to suggest slow pathway conduction. What other important observation can be made?

Commentary: The important observation is that there is atrial activation virtually simultaneous with the ventricular activation after the long A-H interval. This is most compatible with an atrial echo over the AV node (ie, one beat of AV nodal reentry).

The right atrial and right ventricular signals are very useful here since there is no atrial activation on the right ventricular lead and only a tiny far-field ventricular activation on the right atrial lead. Make a mental note of what the A and V components of the EGM look like in sinus rhythm. Then refer back to the EGM in question and compare. This makes the exercise of distinguishing A components from V components easier.

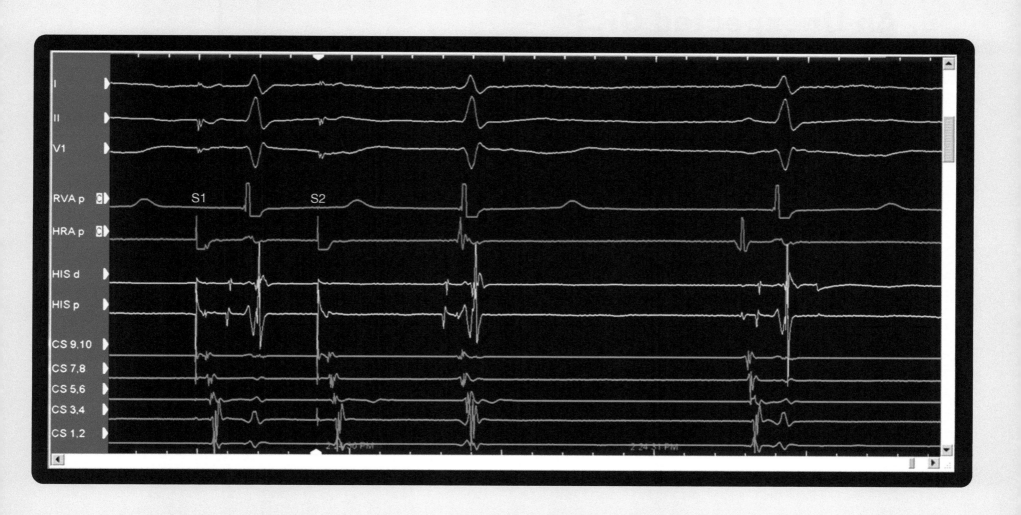

25. An Unexpected QRS

This tracing demonstrates the last two beats of an atrial drive (S1s) and an S2. There is conduction to the QRS after the S2 but then a second QRS follows without any *preceding* atrial activation.

What is the origin of this second unexpected QRS?

Commentary: This unexpected cycle can be a random His extra-systole or can be related to the A signal following the S2. Since the observation was highly reproducible, it is most probably related to the A following S2. This is called a "2 for 1" phenomenon, or "twofer," where the atrial beat after an S2 goes initially over a fast AV nodal pathway with a short PR interval but also goes over a slow AV nodal pathway resulting in two QRS cycles from a single atrial extra-stimulus. You should also note the atrial activation simultaneous with that second QRS (HRA channel). What do you think that would be? It is an AV nodal echo caused by retrograde conduction back up the fast pathway. Hence, the "2 for 1" was followed by an AV nodal echo beat!

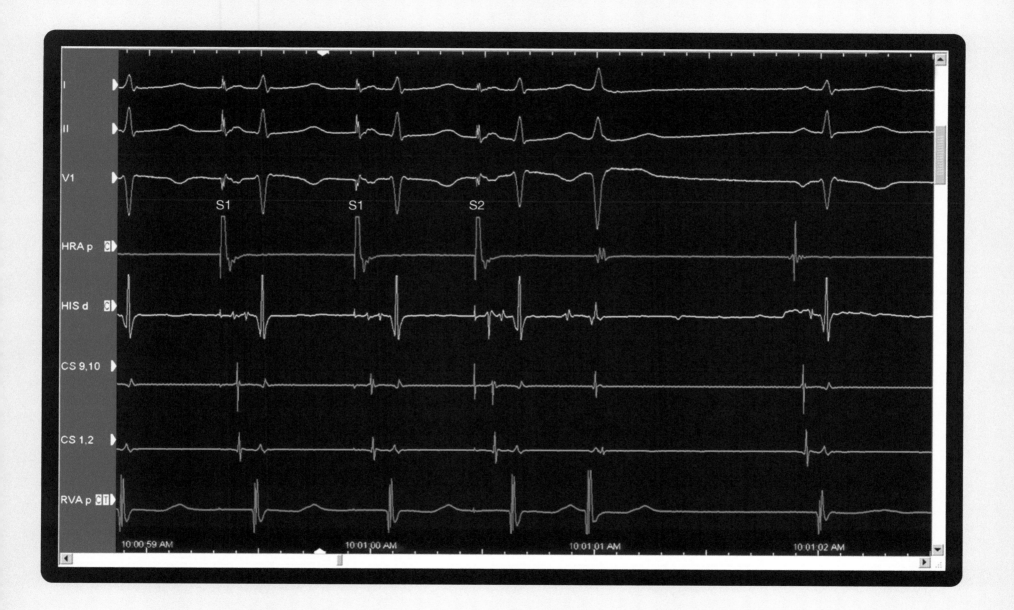

26. Unusual Onset of Tachycardia

In this tracing, we are performing ventricular extra-stimulus pacing with the last two of the S1 drive beats and the S2 shown. After a long pause, a tachycardia starts. What happened?

Commentary: This tachycardia has a normal QRS complex with a normal H-V interval and a nearly simultaneous atrial and ventricular activation. This is in all probability AV nodal reentry (although strictly speaking, we need to see more to definitively rule out the possibility of a junctional tachycardia).

But how did it start? There is no credible atrial activation after the S2, implying that conduction failed to make it to the atrium (blocked). There is a subsequent pause and the sinus node provided an escape cycle (see the early A at the HRA channel just before the QRS). Due to its close proximity to the QRS, it could not have been conducted to the QRS. It then seems reasonable that the QRS is a result of a junctional escape beat.

This then was responsible for setting up AV nodal reentry by several possible mechanisms.

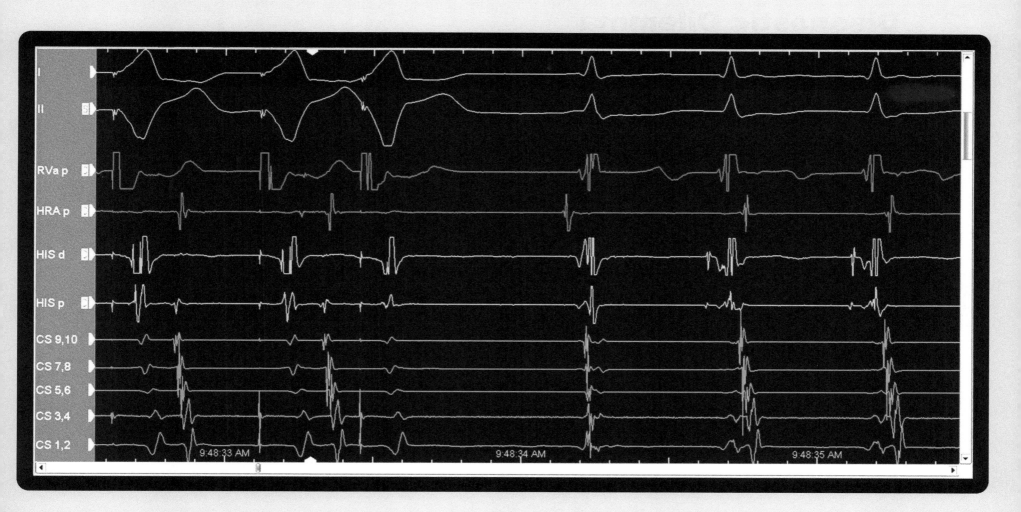

27. Diagnostic Dilemma

This is a common clinical scenario.

This patient had confirmed AVNRT and apparently successful slow pathway ablation. During final testing the finding on this tracing was quite reproducible. We have two junctional beats (beats 4 and 5) following the S1-S2 pacing, the first one occurring 660 msec after the S2.

There are two possible explanations:

1. The S2 blocked and QRS 4 and 5 were junctional escape beats.

2. The S2 conducted over a very slow pathway and initiated two beats of slow AVNRT.

How can we distinguish between these explanations?

Commentary: This is of obvious clinical importance since persistent AV nodal reentry may lead to further ablation while junctional rhythm related to procedural sinus bradycardia will be self-limited and not lead to further intervention.

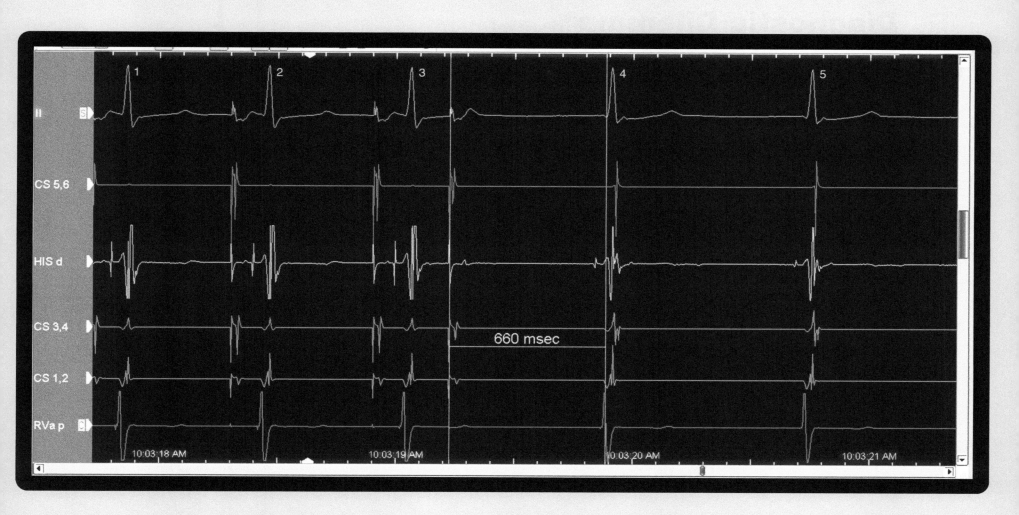

27. **Diagnostic Dilemma** *continued*

We added a third atrial extra-stimulus (S3, the fourth pacing spike) in an attempt to preempt the first junctional beat, which *would have* occurred at the line marked "660 msec."

Did this help distinguish slow AV nodal reentry from junctional rhythm?

Commentary: The S3 conducts to the ventricle with a relatively short A-H interval. This is only compatible with a fully recovered AV node and this would only have occurred if the S2 blocked completely (explanation 1 on page 132) and the next two cycles are junctional.

If it were AV nodal reentry with a long A-H interval (explanation 2 on page 132), the S3 would surely have encountered AV node refractoriness and failed to conduct over the AV node. It would not advance the next QRS; but it did.

It is virtually impossible for a PAC introduced into the cardiac cycle during diastole to advance the subsequent QRS! The S2 would be actually traveling over a very slow pathway. If that is the case, the S3 should not be able to conduct over the AV node since it is "busy" and thus the S3 would be unable to affect the timing of the next V.

Since our S3 advanced the next V, the S2 must have blocked and the diagnosis is explanation 2: junctional escape beats rather than two beats of AVNRT.

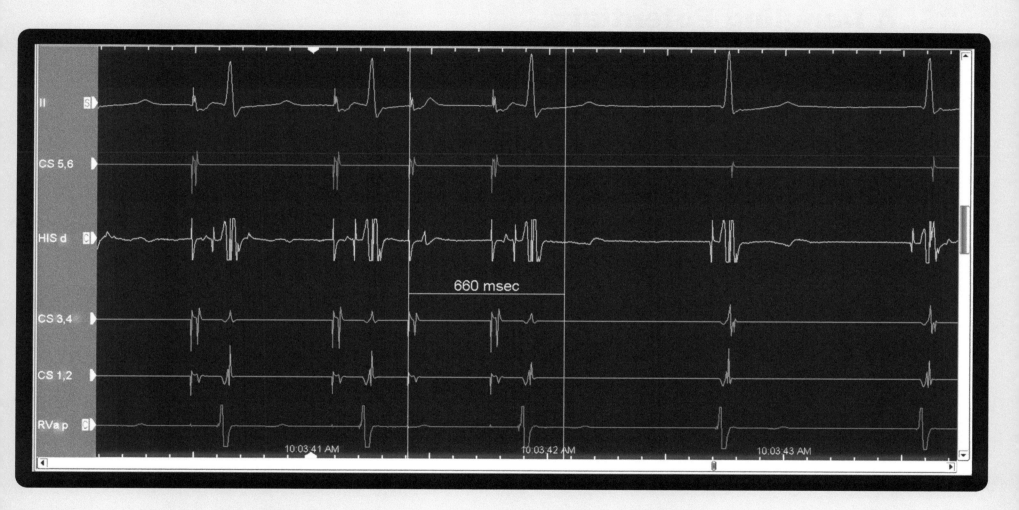

28. A Dangling Potential

This figure, from a patient who was being studied for recurrent SVT, shows the last beat of a ventricular drive (S1) and a closely coupled ventricular extra-stimulus. Atrial activation after the S1 is eccentric, with the distal coronary sinus (CS 3-4) earliest. This is most compatible with a left AP. The S2, however, blocks to the atrium. The observation is reproducible. What is the small deflection after the QRS seen on the HIS d channel? Why is it not seen after the S1?

Commentary: Since the potential is reproducible, it is not random noise. There is no conduction to the atrium so it can't be an atrial deflection. It is most compatible with a retrograde His deflection coming up from the ventricle and, in this case, not able to conduct over the AV node.

It is not seen after the S1 because the HIS deflection is "buried" within the QRS during the normal drive. The extra-stimulus, however, causes conduction delay within the His-Purkinje system and the H comes relatively late after the QRS. It is clearly seen since there is retrograde block over the AP and thus no A to obscure it.

Compare the morphology of the HIS deflections between the retrograde HIS and the antegrade HIS of the following cycle. What difference might you expect between an antegrade and retrograde HIS?

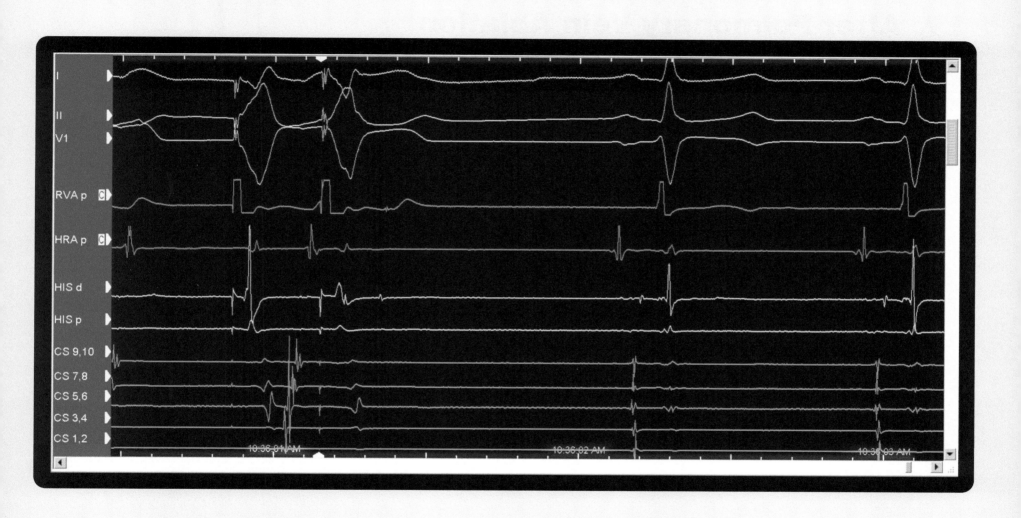

29. After Pulmonary Vein Ablation

This tracing demonstrates pacing from the ablation catheter positioned inside a PV. The multipolar circular catheter (in this instance, Lasso) is also positioned inside the PV. Is this PV isolated?

Commentary: The desired goal of PV ablation is complete block of conduction out of the vein (exit block) and block of conduction into the vein (entrance block). Each stimulus is followed by a near-field EGM in the multipolar (Lasso) catheter indicating capture of the PV musculature inside the PV. These EGMs don't affect the sinus rhythm evident on the surface ECG or the other intracardiac channels. Clearly we have exit block.

In the middle of this tracing, we see a conducted sinus beat. Note that the PV signals are "silent," indicating no conduction into the vein either (entrance block). This vein is now completely isolated.

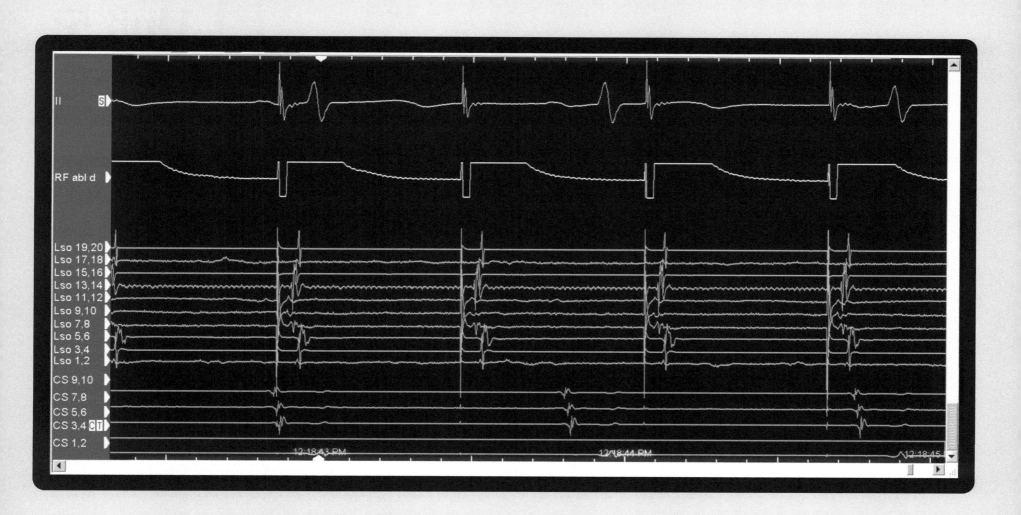

Unit 5:
Cardiac Electrical Axis

In this unit, we will explain cardiac electrical axis and the clinical implications of axis deviations.

There are many excellent publications on ECG analysis and interpretation. However, one topic consistently misunderstood is cardiac electrical axis. It is a concept critical to understanding clinical electrophysiology.

This unit is designed to cut through the complexities of axis determination and simplify your approach towards differentiating normal axis from right or left axis deviations and the clinical implications of such deviations.

A consistent approach to an ECG is essential. The approach I employ is what I call the "RABI" method:

R = Rate and Rhythm
A = Axis
B = Blocks (AV blocks and Bundle Branch Blocks)
I = Ischemia, Injury, and Infarction

In this unit, we will focus on Axis.

UNIT 5 OUTLINE

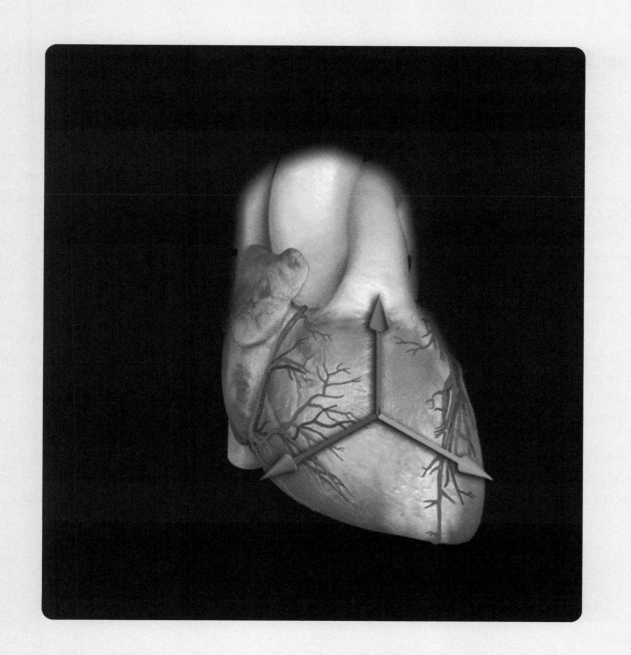

30. Vector Basics

To understand cardiac electrical axis, it is essential to understand vectors. A vector is a graphical representation of the *magnitude* and *direction* of an electrical current.

As an analogy, before buying a car that's parked in the showroom, you look at it from a variety of angles to get a complete 3D picture. The car's position does not change, but your vantage point does. Similarly, the heart's position does not change, but we have the ability to look at it from a variety of angles. This "ability" comes in the form of the 12-lead ECG. The ECG is simply looking at the stationary cardiac vector from a variety of angles.

Hypertrophy increases the magnitude of the vector and pulls it in the direction of the hypertrophy. Infarction on the other hand, decreases the magnitude of the vector and decreases the pull on the vector in the direction of the infarction.

Conduction blocks or delays will change the direction of the vector. If the sequence of ventricular activation is altered due to a delay in a fascicle, the overall electrical axis will be altered.

Vector Principles

Scenario 1: If a wave of depolarization is traveling parallel to and in the same direction as lead 1, you observe a very positive QRS. If the wave is not quite parallel but still in the same general direction as lead 1, the amplitude of the QRS will be reduced, but still positive.

Scenario 2: If a wave of depolarization is traveling parallel, but in the opposite direction to lead 1, you observe a very negative QRS. If the wave is not quite parallel but still generally in the opposite direction to lead 1, the amplitude of the QRS will be reduced but still negative.

Scenario 3: If a wave of depolarization is traveling perpendicular to lead 1, you observe a biphasic QRS. The amplitude of the biphasic deflection varies markedly due, in part, to the gain on the ECG machine.

Commentary: On our EP monitor, we routinely use lead 1, lead 2, and V1. These leads give us 3 dimensions. Lead 1 looks from right to left. Lead 2 looks from superior to inferior. Lead V1 looks from posterior to anterior in the horizontal plane.

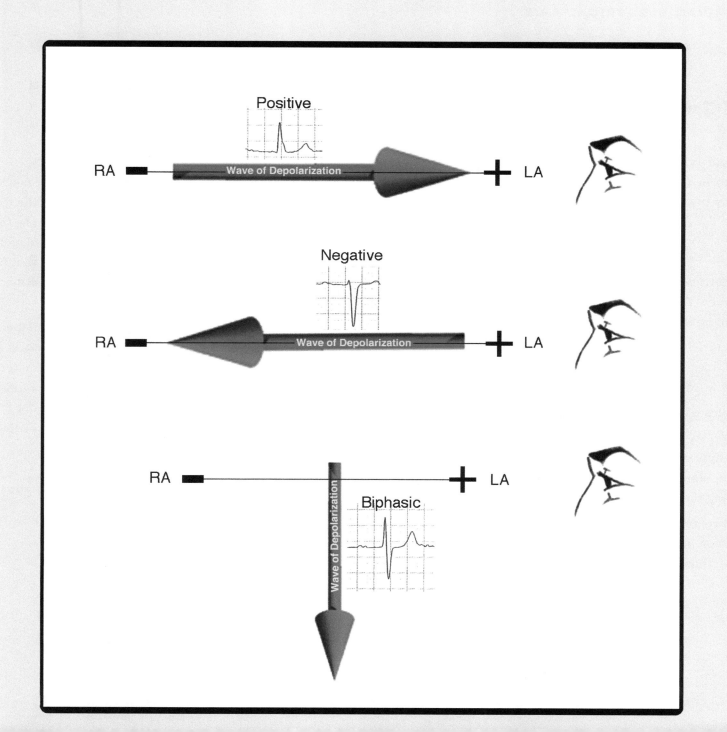

31. Tug-of-War

Cardiac electrical axis is essentially a tug-of-war. Anterior and right-sided forces are in a constant battle with posterior and left-sided forces. As in any tug-of-war, victory may be obtained via one of two options:

Stronger Teammates

1. The right ventricle is anterior in the chest, thus generating anterior forces. The left ventricle is thicker than the RV and posterior to the RV, thus generating stronger forces posteriorly.

2. The right ventricle is also rightward in the chest, thus generating rightward forces. The left ventricle is leftward, thus generating stronger leftward forces.

   Hypertrophies will increase electrical forces (stronger teammates).

   • If the RV hypertrophies (due to pulmonary hypertension or pulmonary stenosis), more rightward forces will be generated, thus pulling the QRS axis toward the right.

   • If the left ventricle hypertrophies (due to systemic hypertension or aortic stenosis), more leftward forces will be generated, thus pulling the ECG axis toward the left.

Weaker Opponents

1. The left bundle branch system has an anterior fascicle and a posterior fascicle. The anterior fascicle pulls the total electrical vector anteriorly. The posterior fascicle pulls the total electrical vector posteriorly. If either fascicle is damaged, delayed, or blocked, the electrical "pull" associated with that fascicle is lost or delayed. This allows the "other side" in this tug-of-war to "win."

Commentary: Axis is not confined to QRS axis. All the same tug-of-war principles apply to the P-wave axis. The P wave is simply smaller! The proximal half of the P wave generally approximates RA depolarization, while the distal half of the P wave represents LA depolarization. Atrial hypertrophy will therefore alter the morphology of the P wave. Examining the P-wave axis helps to establish the origin of an atrial tachycardia.

In the following image, anterior and right-sided forces pull against left and posterior forces.

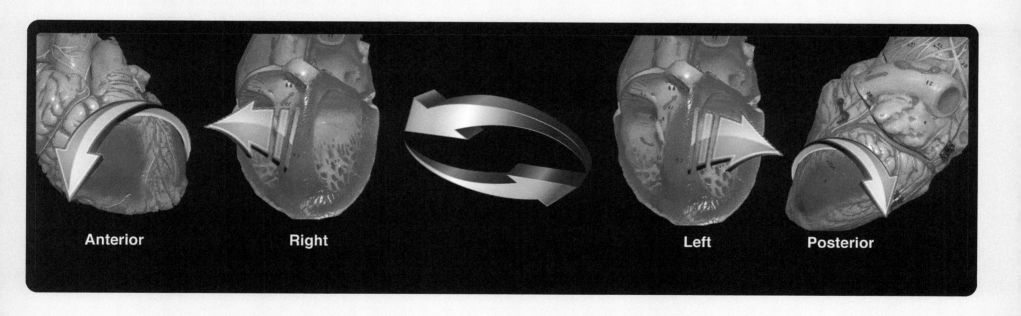

Anterior   Right   Left   Posterior

32. Normal QRS Axis

Let's simplify axis. Normal axis is from −30 to +90 degrees.

Lead 1 and lead 2 are *all* you need to determine axis!

Lead I records electrical activity going right to left. As long as the QRS vector is pointed anywhere leftward, Lead 1 will be positive. If the QRS vector is pointed anywhere to the patient's right, lead 1 will be negative, thus indicating a right axis deviation. If the QRS vector happens to be pointing at exactly 0 degrees, lead 1 will be strongly positive and AVF will be biphasic.

Lead II records electrical activity going from the right arm to the left leg. A QRS vector pointing parallel to and in the same direction as lead II will inscribe a large positive deflection and will be pointing at exactly +60 degrees. If the QRS vector happens to be pointing at exactly −30 degrees, lead 2 will be biphasic. Any vector pointing at greater than −30 degrees will cause lead 2 to be mostly negative, thus indicating LAD.

Commentary: Lead AVF is not helpful when the axis falls between zero degrees and −30 degrees. If the axis points to −20 degrees, AVF will be mostly negative, leading you to believe the patient has a left axis deviation when in fact he/she does not. Left axis deviation starts at −31 degrees or more.

Additionally, it is unnecessary to determine the *EXACT* axis. What *IS* important is to recognize when an axis deviation is present and its clinical implication.

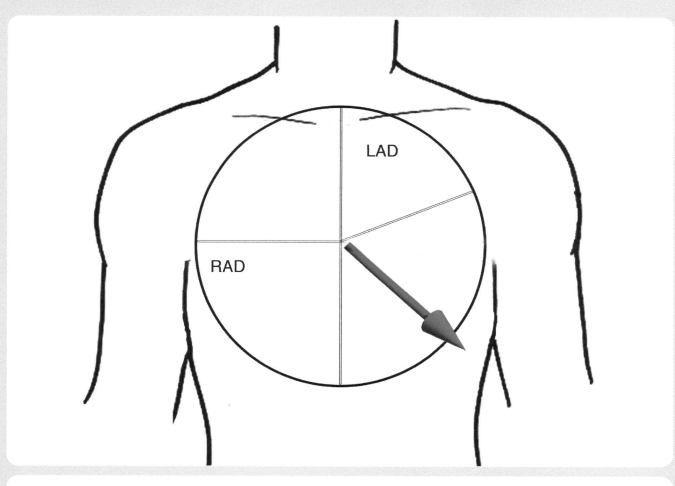

	Normal	LAD	RAD	NW
Lead 1	+	+	-	-
Lead 2	+	-	+	-

32. Normal QRS Axis *continued*

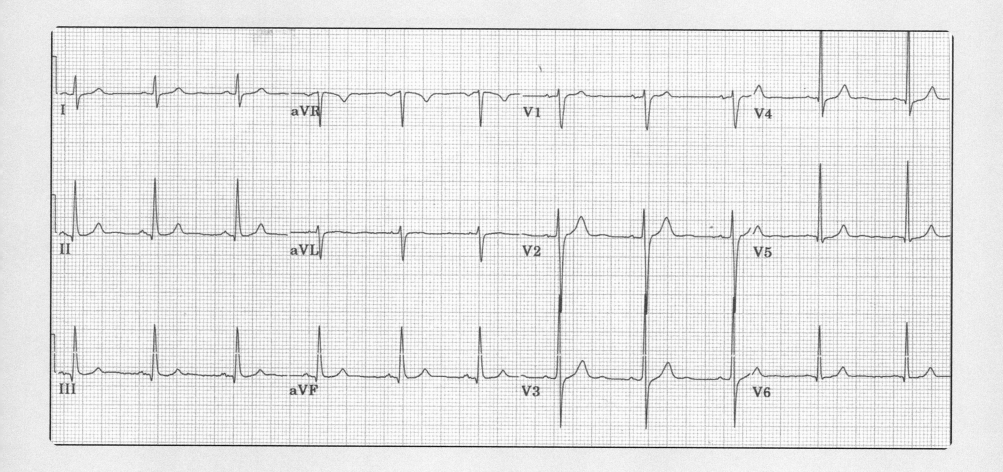

32. Normal QRS Axis *continued*

Commentary: An axis of +90 degrees is within the normal range.

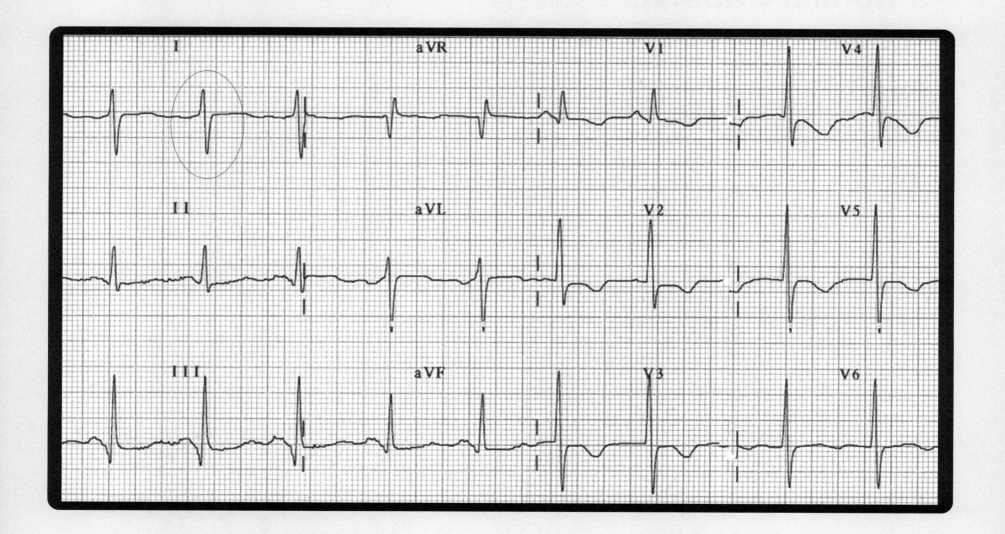

32. Normal QRS Axis *continued*

Commentary: An axis of zero degrees is within the normal range.

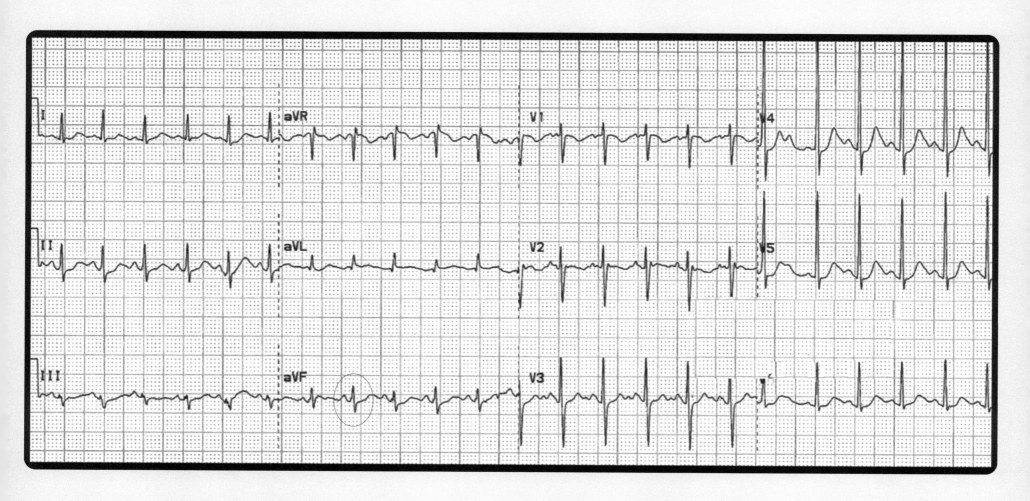

32. Normal QRS Axis *continued*

Commentary: An axis of -30 degrees is within the normal range.

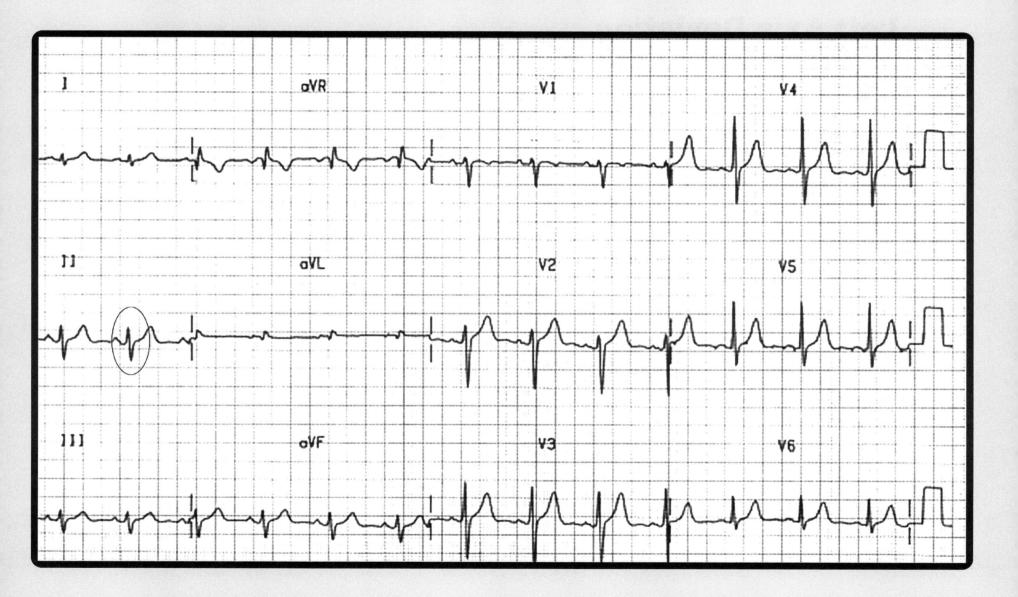

33. Left Axis Deviation

Left ventricular hypertrophy will increasing the electrical pull *toward* the patient's left side causing left axis deviation. Another way to "win" the tug-of-war is to have weaker or injured forces pulling *against* you. Therefore, if you have left anterior hemiblock, those anterior forces are lost leaving the posterior and left-sided forces relatively unopposed, resulting in left axis deviation.

- **Lead 1 is positive.**
- **Lead 2 is negative.**

Aortic stenosis or systemic hypertension will cause left ventricular hypertrophy. Left anterior hemiblock (LAH) may be due to an anterior wall infarction. A hemiblock does not necessarily mean it's pathologically blocked. It may be an indication that depolarization of that fascicle is simply delayed (or late).

Commentary: The differential diagnoses of a left axis deviation are:

- Left ventricular hypertrophy
- Left anterior hemiblock

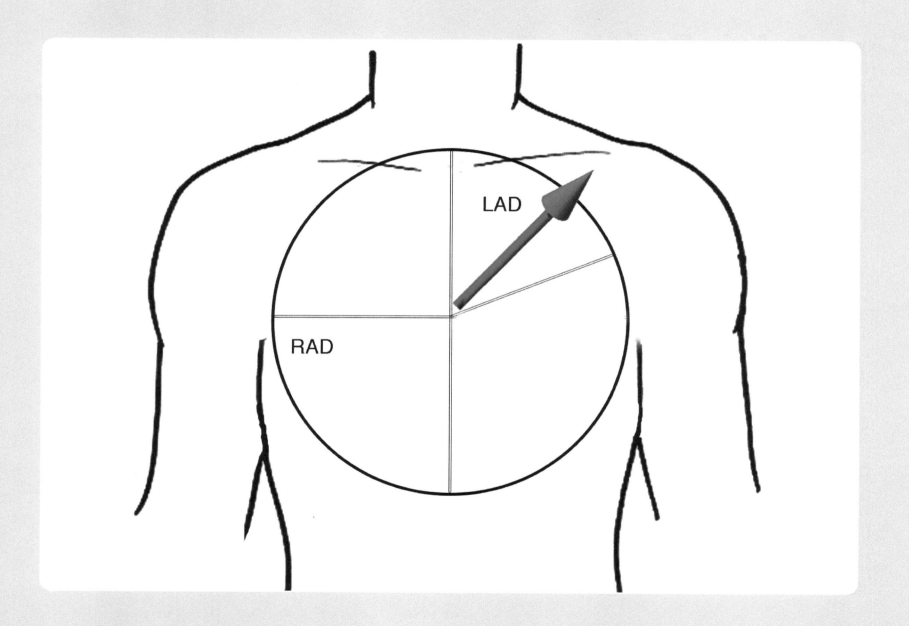

33. Left Axis Deviation *continued*

Commentary: With the loss of anterior forces, the posterior and left forces win the "tug-of-war" resulting in left axis deviation.

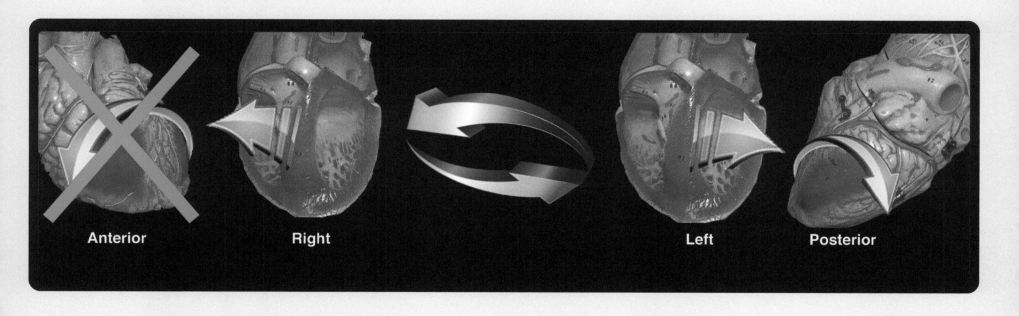

Anterior   **Right**   **Left**   **Posterior**

33. Left Axis Deviation *continued*

Commentary: Notice that the QRS in lead 1 is positive and the QRS in lead 2 is negative.

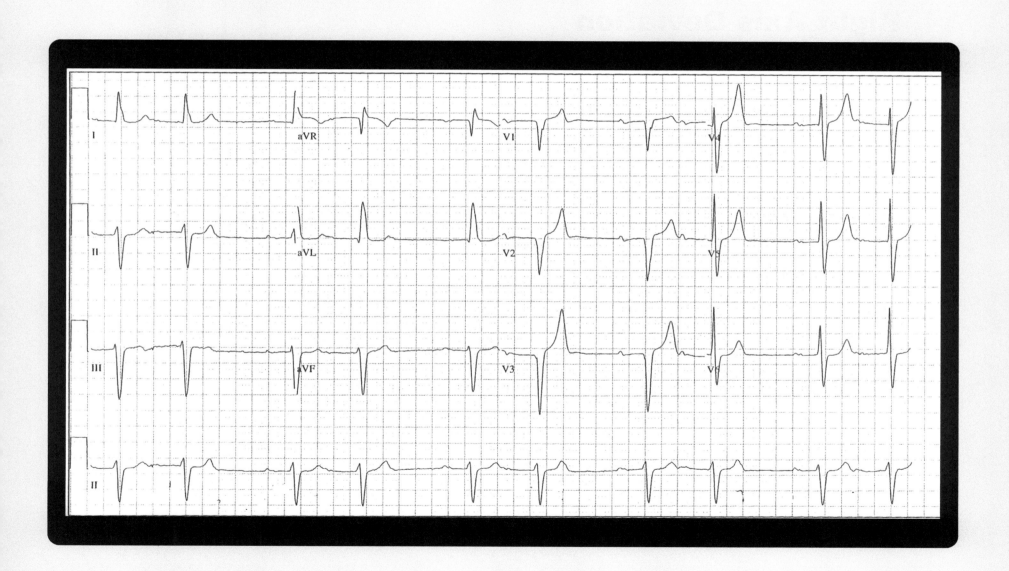

34. Right Axis Deviation

Right ventricular hypertrophy increasing the electrical pull *toward* the patient's right side causing right axis deviation. Another way to win the "tug-of-war" is to have weaker or injured forces pulling *against* you. Therefore, if you have left posterior hemiblock, those posterior forces are lost, leaving the anterior and right-sided forces unopposed, resulting in right axis deviation.

- **Lead 1 is negative.**
- **Lead 2 is positive.**

Pulmonary stenosis or pulmonary hypertension may result in right ventricular hypertrophy. Left posterior hemiblock (LPH) may be due to a more severe anterior wall infarction. Again, hemiblocks may be nothing more than an indication that depolarization of that fascicle is late

Commentary: The differential diagnoses of a right axis deviation are:

- Right ventricular hypertrophy
- Left posterior hemiblock

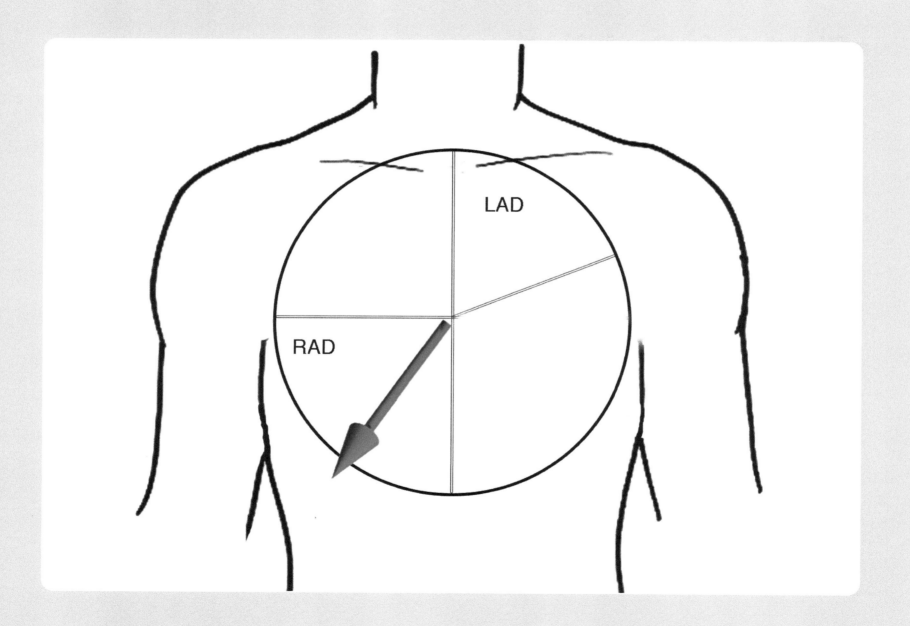

34. Right Axis Deviation *continued*

Commentary: With the loss of posterior forces, the anterior and right forces win the "tug-of-war" resulting in right axis deviation.

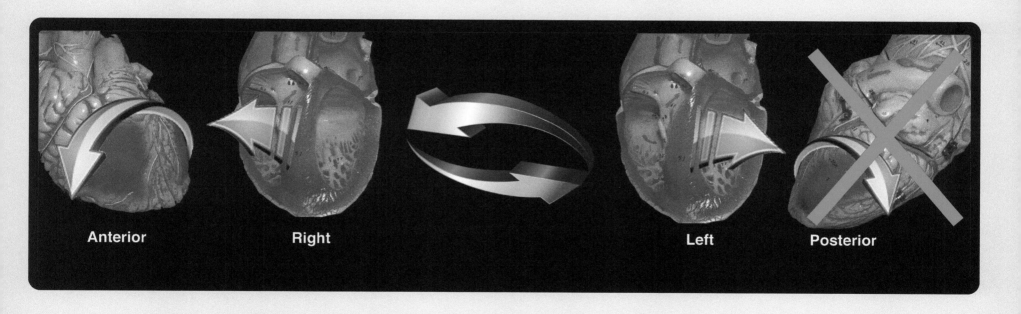

Anterior   Right   Left   Posterior

34. Right Axis Deviation *continued*

Commentary: Notice that the QRS in lead 1 is negative and the QRS in lead 2 is positive.

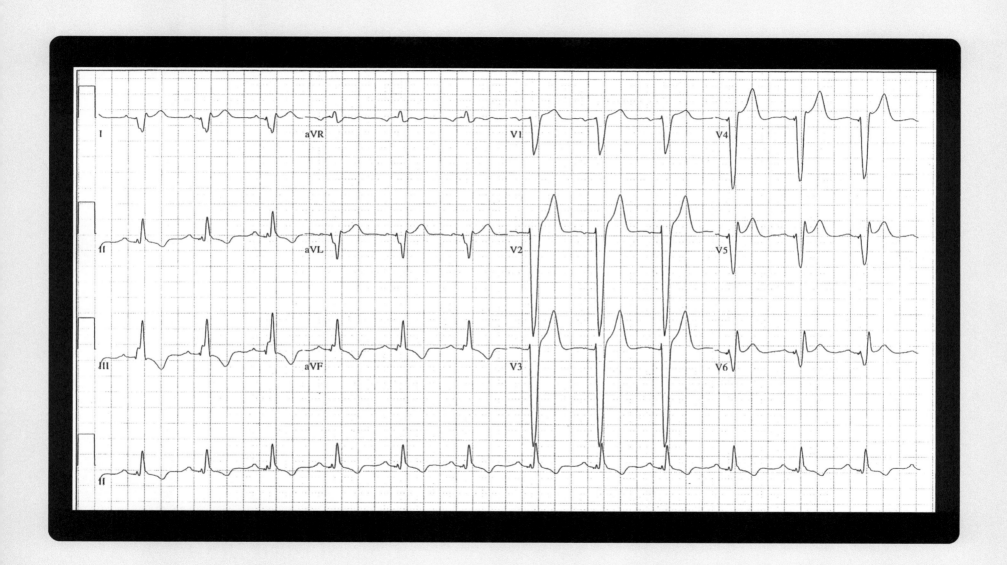

35. North–West Axis

A very unusual axis is often referred to as a north–west axis. This is diagnosed by:

- **Lead 1 is negative.**
- **Lead 2 is negative.**

This is an axis usually seen during LV VT. Since it is originating in the LV:

1. The ECG will also display an atypical RBBB pattern. This is because the left bundle system is activated early, and thus the right bundle system is activated late. The right bundle is simply late, not pathologically blocked.

2. As shown in the graphic on the right, if the wave of depolarization originates in the left ventricular apex, it must spread left to right (lead 1 negative) and low to high (lead 2 negative), thus generating a north-west axis.

Commentary: The differential diagnosis of a north-west axis is:

- LV VT

If the LV VT originates near the anterior aspect of the mitral valve (basal origin) lead 2 may be positive, indicating "high-to-low" depolarization, and thus you will not see a north-west axis.

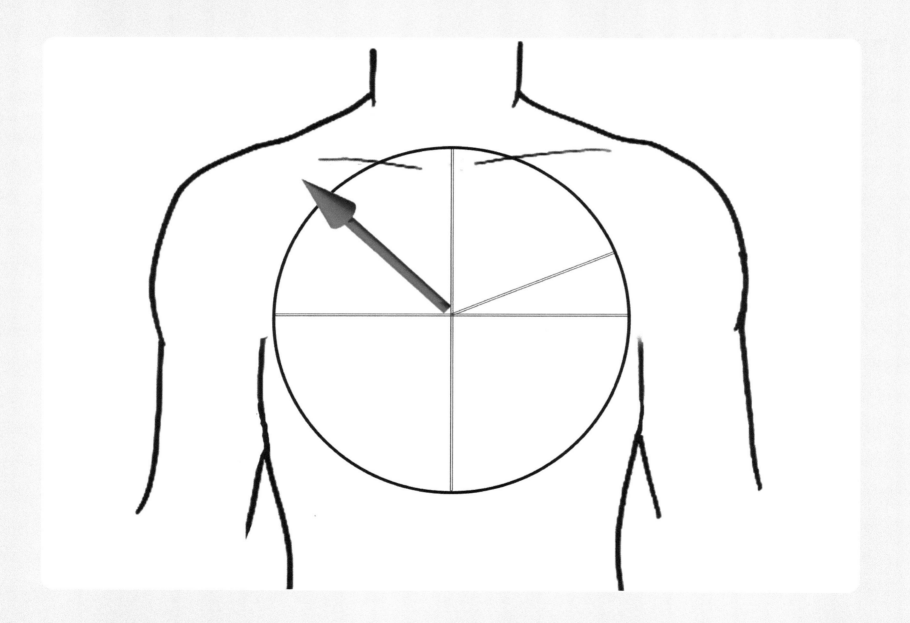

35. **North–West Axis** *continued*

Commentary: Notice that the QRS in lead 1 is negative and the QRS in lead 2 is negative and a RBBB pattern. The RBBB pattern is not a "typical" RBBB pattern. This example indicates that the right bundle branch is simply "late," not pathologically blocked.

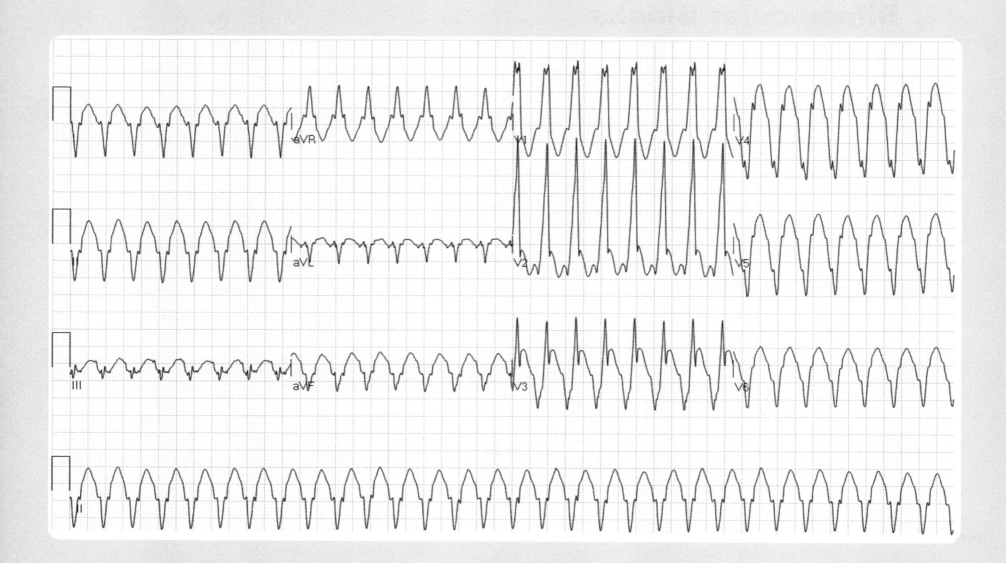

36. Bifascicular Blocks

It is not unusual to have delay or block in more than one fascicle.

Here are three examples:

Tracing #1: Lead 2 is negative, indicating left anterior hemiblock (LAH). That's one fascicle. Lead V1 is positive, indicating a "typical" right bundle branch block. That's the second fascicle. The only fascicle that is still conducting normally is the left posterior fascicle.

Commentary: Hemiblocks do not necessarily imply pathological damage. Any of the fascicles of the conduction system (right bundle, left anterior fascicle, and left posterior fascicle) may be simply depolarized "late."

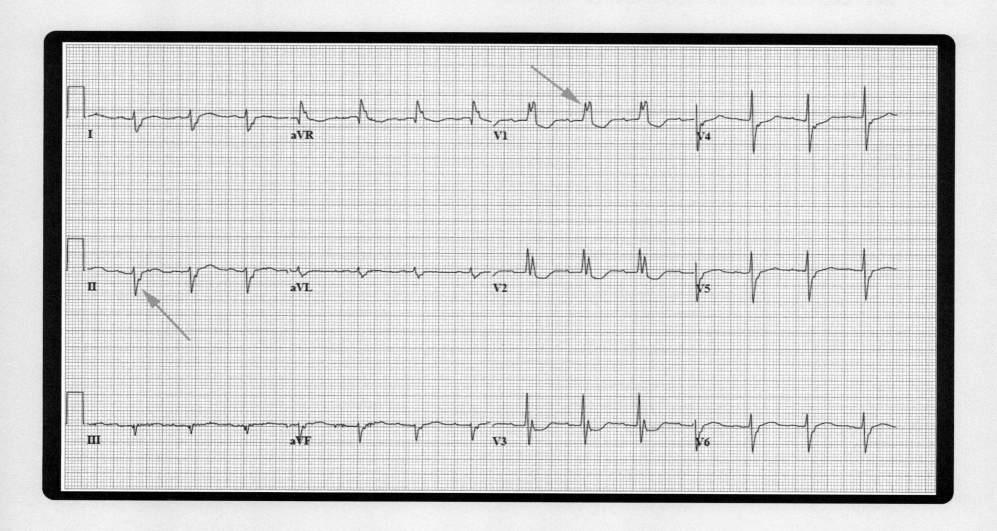

36. **Bifascicular Blocks** *continued*

Tracing #2: Lead 1 is negative, indicating a left posterior hemiblock (LPH). That's one fascicle. Lead V1 is positive, indicating right bundle branch block. That's the second fascicle. However, in this example, the RBBB is not "typical." This implies that the right bundle is simply "late," not necessarily "blocked." Since the right bundle is late and the posterior fascicle is blocked (or late), we can infer that the only fascicle conducting normally is the left anterior fascicle.

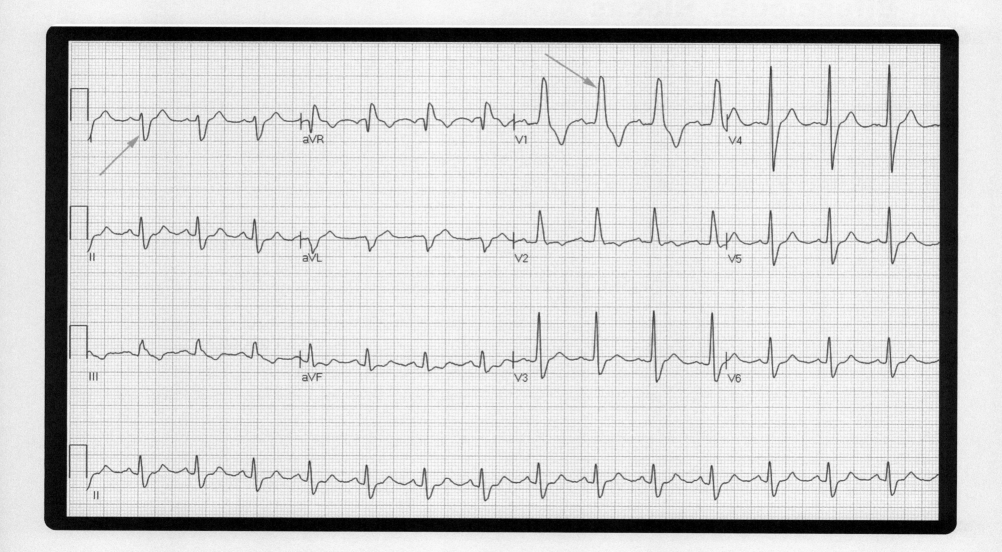

36. **Bifascicular Blocks** *continued*

Tracing #3: Lead 2 is negative, indicating left anterior hemiblock (LAH). Lead V1 is positive, indicating right bundle branch block. Again, this is not a "typical" RBBB pattern. This implies that the right bundle is being depolarized "late."

This tracing is actually VT originating in the LV (a RBBB pattern) and posteriorly, somewhere close to the left posterior fascicle; therefore, the left anterior fascicle is late (LAH).

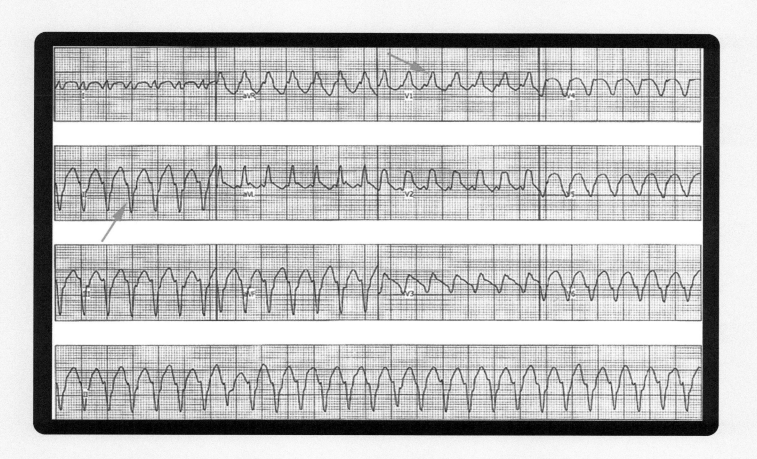